# FUNDAMENTAL WEIGHT TRAINING

## David Sandler

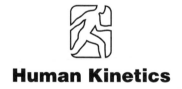

**Human Kinetics**

**Library of Congress Cataloging-in-Publication Data**

Sandler, David.
  Fundamental weight training / David Sandler.
     p. cm.
  ISBN-13: 978-0-7360-8280-8 (soft cover)
  ISBN-10: 0-7360-8280-8 (soft cover)
  1. Weight training. I. Title.
  GV546.B87 2010
  613.7'13--dc22

                              2009052430
ISBN-10: 0-7360-8280-8 (print)
ISBN-13: 978-0-7360-8280-8 (print)

This publication is written and published to provide accurate and authoritative information relevant to the subject matter presented. It is published and sold with the understanding that the author and publisher are not engaged in rendering legal, medical, or other professional services by reason of their authorship or publication of this work. If medical or other expert assistance is required, the services of a competent professional person should be sought.

Illustrations on pages xi and xii are reprinted, by permission, from National Strength and Conditioning Association, 2008, *Essentials of strength training and conditioning,* 3rd ed. (Champaign, IL: Human Kinetics), 68.

This book is a revised edition of *Weight Training Fundamentals*, published in 2003 by Human Kinetics.

**Acquisitions Editor:** Justin Klug; **Developmental Editor:** Heather Healy; **Assistant Editor:** Michael Bishop; **Copyeditor:** Patricia MacDonald; **Graphic Designer:** Joe Buck; **Graphic Artist:** Francine Hamerski; **Cover Designer:** Keith Blomberg; **Photographer (cover and interior):** Neil Bernstein; **Visual Production Assistant:** Joyce Brumfield; **Photo Production Manager:** Jason Allen; **Art Manager:** Kelly Hendren; **Associate Art Manager:** Alan L. Wilborn; **Illustrators:** Andrew Recher (anatomy illustrations on pages xi and xii) and Alan L. Wilborn (figure 15.1); **Printer:** United Graphics

We thank Bodysport in Summerlin/Las Vegas, Nevada for assistance in providing the location for the photo shoot for this book. We thank the models: Ashley Klemz, Courtney Hayes, Johnathan Samokhvalov, Martin Morales, Chris Henderson, Kylie Wassel.

Human Kinetics books are available at special discounts for bulk purchase. Special editions or book excerpts can also be created to specification. For details, contact the Special Sales Manager at Human Kinetics.

Printed in the United States of America    10 9 8 7 6 5 4 3 2 1

The paper in this book is certified under a sustainable forestry program.

**Human Kinetics**
Web site: www.HumanKinetics.com

*United States:* Human Kinetics
P.O. Box 5076
Champaign, IL 61825-5076
800-747-4457
e-mail: humank@hkusa.com

*Canada:* Human Kinetics
475 Devonshire Road Unit 100
Windsor, ON N8Y 2L5
800-465-7301 (in Canada only)
e-mail: info@hkcanada.com

*Europe:* Human Kinetics
107 Bradford Road
Stanningley
Leeds LS28 6AT, United Kingdom
+44 (0) 113 255 5665
e-mail: hk@hkeurope.com

*Australia:* Human Kinetics
57A Price Avenue
Lower Mitcham, South Australia 5062
08 8372 0999
e-mail: info@hkaustralia.com

*New Zealand:* Human Kinetics
P.O. Box 80
Torrens Park, South Australia 5062
0800 222 062
e-mail: info@hknewzealand.com

E4797

For my wife, Debbie, whose tireless efforts to support my crazy ideas have allowed me to learn, teach, and practice my craft. And for my son, Jack, you are my inspiration to be the best I can at whatever I do. I love you both very much!

# CONTENTS

Exercise Finder   vi
Acknowledgments   x
Key to Muscles   xi

CHAPTER 1
**Introduction to Weight Training** . . . . . . .1

CHAPTER 2
**Weight Room Language and Protocol** . . .7

CHAPTER 3
**Types of Resistance Training** . . . . . . . 17

CHAPTER 4
**Warm Up, Stretch, Cool Down** . . . . . . 35

CHAPTER 5
**Chest** . . . . . . . . . . . . . . . . . . . . 51

CHAPTER 6
**Back** . . . . . . . . . . . . . . . . . . . . . 63

CHAPTER 7
**Shoulders** . . . . . . . . . . . . . . . . . . 77

CHAPTER 8
**Traps** . . . . . . . . . . . . . . . . . . . . 87

CHAPTER 9

**Arms** . . . . . . . . . . . . . **95**

CHAPTER 10

**Core** . . . . . . . . . . . . .**119**

CHAPTER 11

**Glutes and Hips** . . . . . . . . **139**

CHAPTER 12

**Quads** . . . . . . . . . . . . **151**

CHAPTER 13

**Hamstrings**. . . . . . . . . . **163**

CHAPTER 14

**Lower Legs**. . . . . . . . . . **173**

CHAPTER 15

**Program Design** . . . . . . . . **185**

CHAPTER 16

**Sample Programs** . . . . . . . **197**

**About the Author   211**

# EXERCISE FINDER

| Exercise | Target area | | | | | | | | | | Page no. |
|---|---|---|---|---|---|---|---|---|---|---|---|
| | Chest | Back | Shoulders | Traps | Arms | Core | Glutes and hips | Quads | Hamstrings | Lower legs | |
| **Static stretches** | | | | | | | | | | | |
| Biceps stretch | | | | | ✓ | | | | | | 43 |
| Calf stretch | | | | | | | | | | ✓ | 39 |
| Groin stretch | | | | | | | ✓ | | ✓ | | 40 |
| Hamstring and lower back stretch | | ✓ | | | | | | | ✓ | | 40 |
| Hip flexor stretch | | | | | | | ✓ | ✓ | | | 41 |
| Pec stretch | ✓ | | ✓ | | | | | | | | 41 |
| Quadriceps stretch | | | | | | | | ✓ | | | 39 |
| Rear deltoid and upper back stretch | | ✓ | ✓ | ✓ | | | | | | | 42 |
| Triceps stretch | | | | | ✓ | | | | | | 42 |
| Upper back stretch | | ✓ | | ✓ | | | | | | | 43 |
| **Dynamic stretches** | | | | | | | | | | | |
| Chain breakers | ✓ | ✓ | ✓ | ✓ | | | | | | | 45 |
| Duck walk | | | | | | | ✓ | ✓ | ✓ | ✓ | 46 |
| Knee-to-chest walk | | | | | | | ✓ | ✓ | ✓ | ✓ | 45 |
| Lateral push-up walk | ✓ | | ✓ | | ✓ | ✓ | | | | | 48 |
| Lunge and reach | ✓ | | | | | ✓ | ✓ | ✓ | ✓ | ✓ | 44 |
| Mountain climbers | | | | | | ✓ | ✓ | ✓ | ✓ | ✓ | 48 |
| Overhead squat | ✓ | | | | | ✓ | ✓ | ✓ | | ✓ | 47 |
| Spider-man | ✓ | ✓ | | | | ✓ | ✓ | ✓ | ✓ | ✓ | 49 |
| Stationary inchworm | ✓ | ✓ | | | | ✓ | ✓ | | ✓ | ✓ | 47 |
| Trunk rotations | | | | | | ✓ | ✓ | | | | 46 |
| **Machine-based strength** | | | | | | | | | | | |
| Adductor cable lift | | | | | | | ✓ | | ✓ | | 146 |
| Back extension | | | | | | ✓ | | | ✓ | | 122 |
| Cable cross | ✓ | | ✓ | | | | | | | | 60 |
| Cable curl | | | | | ✓ | | | | | | 104 |
| Cable (or machine) pec fly | ✓ | | ✓ | | | | | | | | 58 |
| Cable reverse-grip triceps pull-down | | | | | ✓ | | | | | | 113 |

| Exercise | Target area | | | | | | | | | | Page no. |
|---|---|---|---|---|---|---|---|---|---|---|---|
| | Chest | Back | Shoulders | Traps | Arms | Core | Glutes and hips | Quads | Hamstrings | Lower legs | |
| **Machine-based strength** *(continued)* | | | | | | | | | | | |
| Front pull | | ✓ | | ✓ | ✓ | | | | | | 69 |
| Hip extension | | | | | | | ✓ | | ✓ | | 143 |
| Hip flexor cable lift | | | | | | | ✓ | ✓ | | | 147 |
| Lat pull-down | | ✓ | | ✓ | ✓ | | | | | | 67 |
| Leg extension | | | | | | | | ✓ | | | 157 |
| Leg press | | | | | | | ✓ | ✓ | | | 140 |
| Leg press heel raise | | | | | | | | | | ✓ | 176 |
| Low-cable kickback | | | | | | | ✓ | | ✓ | | 144 |
| Lying leg curl | | | | | | | | | ✓ | | 164 |
| Scapular retraction | | ✓ | | ✓ | | | | | | | 92 |
| Seated calf heel raise | | | | | | | | | | ✓ | 178 |
| Seated leg curl | | | | | | | | | ✓ | | 166 |
| Seated row | | ✓ | | ✓ | ✓ | | | | | | 64 |
| Side-cable lift | | | | | | | ✓ | | | | 145 |
| Single-leg curl | | | | | | | | | ✓ | | 167 |
| Straight-arm pull-down | | ✓ | | ✓ | ✓ | | | | | | 71 |
| Triceps push-down | | | | | ✓ | | | | | | 98 |
| **Dumbbell strength** | | | | | | | | | | | |
| Dumbbell bench press | ✓ | | ✓ | | ✓ | | | | | | 55 |
| Dumbbell curl | | | | | ✓ | | | | | | 96 |
| Dumbbell pec fly | ✓ | | ✓ | | | | | | | | 59 |
| Dumbbell pullover | ✓ | ✓ | | | | | | | | | 70 |
| Dumbbell row | | ✓ | | ✓ | ✓ | | | | | | 66 |
| Dumbbell squat | | | | | ✓ | ✓ | ✓ | ✓ | | | 156 |
| Dumbbell triceps kickback | | | | | ✓ | | | | | | 111 |
| Front raise | | | ✓ | ✓ | | | | | | | 81 |
| Isolated dumbbell curl | | | | | ✓ | | | | | | 102 |
| Lateral raise | | | ✓ | ✓ | | | | | | | 82 |
| Lunge | | | | | | | ✓ | ✓ | ✓ | ✓ | 158 |
| Overhead triceps extension | | | | | ✓ | | | | | | 112 |

*(continued)*

Exercise Finder  *(continued)*

| Exercise | Chest | Back | Shoulders | Traps | Arms | Core | Glutes and hips | Quads | Hamstrings | Lower legs | Page no. |
|---|---|---|---|---|---|---|---|---|---|---|---|
| **Dumbbell strength (continued)** | | | | | | | | | | | |
| Rear deltoid fly | | | ✓ | ✓ | | | | | | | 83 |
| Shoulder press | | | ✓ | | ✓ | | | | | | 78 |
| Side bend | | | | | | ✓ | | | | | 125 |
| Single-arm bench press | ✓ | | ✓ | | ✓ | | | | | | 56 |
| Supine triceps extension | | | | | ✓ | | | | | | 107 |
| Unstable bench press | ✓ | | ✓ | | ✓ | | | | | | 57 |
| Wrist curl | | | | | ✓ | | | | | | 100 |
| **Barbell strength** | | | | | | | | | | | |
| Barbell shoulder press | | | ✓ | | ✓ | | | | | | 80 |
| Bench press | ✓ | | ✓ | | ✓ | | | | | | 52 |
| Bent-over barbell row | | ✓ | | ✓ | ✓ | | | | | | 72 |
| Close-grip bench press | ✓ | | ✓ | | ✓ | | | | | | 110 |
| Front squat | | | ✓ | | | ✓ | ✓ | ✓ | | ✓ | 154 |
| Incline bench press | ✓ | | ✓ | | ✓ | | | | | | 54 |
| Preacher curl | | | | | ✓ | | | | | | 105 |
| Reverse-grip barbell curl | | | | | ✓ | | | | | | 106 |
| Romanian deadlift | | | | | | ✓ | ✓ | | ✓ | | 128 |
| Shoulder shrug | | | | ✓ | | | | | | | 88 |
| Single-leg squat | | | | | | ✓ | ✓ | ✓ | | ✓ | 155 |
| Squat | | | | | | ✓ | ✓ | ✓ | | ✓ | 152 |
| Straight bar curl | | | | | ✓ | | | | | | 103 |
| Supine triceps extension | | | | | ✓ | | | | | | 107 |
| Upright row | | | ✓ | ✓ | | | | | | | 90 |
| Wrist curl | | | | | ✓ | | | | | | 100 |
| **Body-weight strength** | | | | | | | | | | | |
| Bench dip | ✓ | | ✓ | | ✓ | | | | | | 109 |
| Chin-up | | ✓ | | ✓ | ✓ | | | | | | 68 |
| Crunch | | | | | | ✓ | | | | | 120 |
| Dip | ✓ | | ✓ | | ✓ | | | | | | 108 |
| Elbow to hand plank lift | ✓ | | | | ✓ | ✓ | | | | | 131 |
| Fire hydrant and rotational fire hydrant | | | | | | | ✓ | ✓ | | | 129 |

| Exercise | Target area | | | | | | | | | | Page no. |
|---|---|---|---|---|---|---|---|---|---|---|---|
| | Chest | Back | Shoulders | Traps | Arms | Core | Glutes and hips | Quads | Hamstrings | Lower legs | |
| **Body-weight strength** *(continued)* | | | | | | | | | | | |
| Heel raise | | | | | | | | | | ✓ | 174 |
| Lateral plank raise | ✓ | | | | ✓ | ✓ | | | | | 132 |
| Plank | ✓ | | | | ✓ | ✓ | | | | | 130 |
| Pelvic raise | | | | | | ✓ | | | | | 126 |
| Reverse crunch | | | | | | ✓ | | | | | 127 |
| Single-leg heel raise | | | | | | | | | | ✓ | 177 |
| Single-leg squat | | | | | | ✓ | ✓ | ✓ | | ✓ | 155 |
| Squat heel raise | | | | | | | | | | | 179 |
| Stability ball leg curl | | | | | | | ✓ | | ✓ | ✓ | 169 |
| Step-up | | ✓ | | | | ✓ | ✓ | ✓ | ✓ | ✓ | 142 |
| Superman | | ✓ | | | | ✓ | ✓ | | | | 133 |
| Twisting crunch | | | | | | ✓ | | | | | 124 |
| Walking lunge | | | | | | ✓ | ✓ | ✓ | ✓ | ✓ | 159 |
| **Resistance tubing, partner, and other methods** | | | | | | | | | | | |
| Ankle inversion and eversion | | | | | | | | | | ✓ | 181 |
| Axe chop | | ✓ | ✓ | ✓ | ✓ | ✓ | ✓ | | ✓ | | 135 |
| Scarecrow row | | ✓ | | ✓ | | ✓ | | | | | 91 |
| Standing rotational twist | | | | | | ✓ | ✓ | | | | 134 |
| Toe pull | | | | | | | | | | ✓ | 180 |
| Wrist roller | | | | | ✓ | | | | | | 114 |

# ACKNOWLEDGMENTS

To make a list of all those who have impacted my life and contributed to my learning would be a futile effort, and some people would inevitably be unintentionally left out. Rather, I would like to acknowledge all of the students I have had the pleasure of teaching, all of the athletes I have had the joy of coaching, and the clients I have had the opportunity to train. Without you and your hard work, this book would never have materialized, as your enthusiasm motivated me to find a better way. I would also like to thank the schools I have learned from and taught at. Knowledge is simply a vehicle—without fuel, it won't work. You have taught me how to turn water into gasoline, and I am forever indebted.

I would also like to thank all of the teams, media production companies, equipment manufacturers, magazines, certification organizations, and sponsors for inviting me in to join in your triumphs and allowing me to learn and grow with the diverse and constantly changing fields of health, fitness, and sports performance. I wish to separately express my sincere gratitude to the world's largest sports and fitness weekend event co-founders, Jim Lorimer and its namesake Arnold Schwarzenegger and their family that is collectively known as The Arnold Sports Festival, for bringing fitness to the world and believing in my ability to lead your educational efforts.

And lastly, on behalf of my brother, Mike, and sister, Lori, I want to thank our parents, Joyce and Steve, for their incredible support and never-ending patience with everything we have tried to do.

# KEY TO MUSCLES

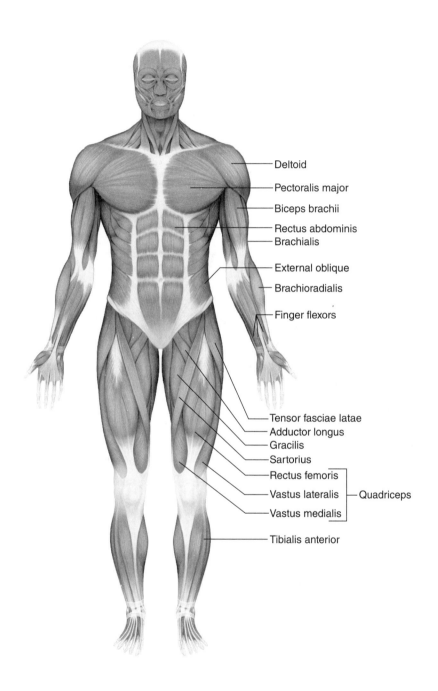

- Deltoid
- Pectoralis major
- Biceps brachii
- Rectus abdominis
- Brachialis
- External oblique
- Brachioradialis
- Finger flexors
- Tensor fasciae latae
- Adductor longus
- Gracilis
- Sartorius
- Rectus femoris
- Vastus lateralis
- Vastus medialis
- Tibialis anterior

Quadriceps

*(continued)*

## Key to Muscles *(continued)*

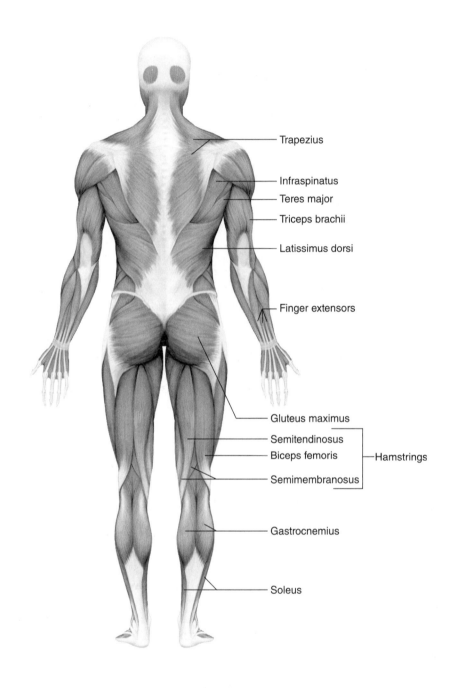

Trapezius

Infraspinatus

Teres major

Triceps brachii

Latissimus dorsi

Finger extensors

Gluteus maximus

Semitendinosus

Biceps femoris — Hamstrings

Semimembranosus

Gastrocnemius

Soleus

# 1

# INTRODUCTION TO WEIGHT TRAINING

Good, you've decided to begin a weight training program. You've made the right move by choosing to do it properly. When exercises are performed correctly, resistance training can have terrific results, such as increasing strength, power, and muscular endurance; improving balance and coordination; and decreasing body fat. When poor technique is used, however, or no attention is paid to proper form, resistance training can lead to injury.

For most people, exercise presents many challenges, and adding a weight training program makes the task even harder. You've already completed the first step by picking up this book—you've chosen to get started! So now it is time to take control of your body and get in shape, not only to look and feel good but also to be able to perform both normal daily tasks and athletic movements.

Embrace weights and they will reward you far more than any other form of exercise can. Increase muscle density, and you will burn more calories. Increase muscle appearance, and you will feel better about yourself. Increase muscle size and endurance, and just about everything you do, such as walking up a flight of stairs, will feel easier. It is a win–win situation when weight training is part of your life.

## WEIGHT TRAINING BASICS

Much of the lore surrounding weight training is based on modern principles from bodybuilding; early weight training dates back thousands of years, when humans were not only performing feats of strength but also training for them. However, it is only in the last two decades that we have come to realize that weight training can promote health and well-being. Because of its long and varied history, if you try to search for a single definition of weight training, you will find many. If you try to search for a single philosophy of weight training, you will find many. And if you try to search for a single program that can match your needs, well, good luck, because you will find thousands!

Additionally, a number of common myths surround weight training, including that it is dangerous, reduces flexibility, and can stunt growth. However, research has proven time and again not only that those statements are false but also that the opposite may be true. In fact, weight training is one of the safest forms of physical activity, having a much lower injury rate than other common recreational activities like basketball, tennis, golf, or running. As long as you follow some simple guidelines, your weight training experience can be injury free.

Moreover, weight training can help prevent injuries that can be caused by other sports and activities. Whether you are playing a sport or walking on an icy street, injuries can occur at any time. Stronger bones, muscles, joints, and connective tissue will make you more resistant to the acute injuries that occur during falls or during collisions with opponents, but the real benefits of weight training come in the prevention of the chronic shoulder, knee, and back pain that can make everyday life more difficult.

Muscle imbalances resulting from undertraining or overuse appear to be a common cause of injury. Most sports and many of our daily activities force us into a position where one side of the body is used more than the other, leading to muscle imbalances. Muscle imbalances cause the body to move incorrectly, resulting in excessive strain on some muscles and joints. Some studies have noted that a muscle imbalance of greater than 10 percent between the right and left sides of the body increases the risk of injury by 20 times. Training the right and left sides separately using resistance tubing, dumbbells, and unilateral machines, which allow for each limb to move individually, can correct many of these imbalances and decrease your risk of developing chronic injuries and aches. But in general, a full-body weight training program will certainly reduce your risk of injury.

Since many people assume weight training "bulks you up," it is often neglected, misunderstood, and when finally applied, done incorrectly. Weight training alone will not increase muscle size significantly (known as hypertrophy) unless you are on a program that applies specific techniques and principles for building muscle. This is good news for those looking to use weight training for health reasons but who do not wish to bulk up. Weight training can be used to improve muscular endurance, which tends to produce a more slender look and provide more regularly usable strength for everyday tasks, such as walking or yard work. If you are interested in improving your sport performance, weight training can improve strength and power, giving you that added edge over your opponents. In any case, everyone should engage in physical activity that includes a weight training program. But again, to see these specific results, your program must be designed to match your goals.

To understand the value of weight training, it is necessary to understand how the body works. The human body is more complex than any machine ever built, and it may be impossible to understand it completely. Over the past 100 years, research has unveiled some pretty cool stuff about the overall benefits of weight training, and we have come to better understand why our bodies increase in size, strength, and power when using external loads for resistance.

We know that when we weight train, we place a stress on the specific muscle being used, which causes microdamage to the muscle's internal structures (e.g., the protein filaments myosin, actin, troponin, and tropomyosin). With adequate rest and nutrition, the damage is not only repaired to withstand the same stress but also fortified to battle even greater stresses. This was scientifically proven in the early 1920s when a physician by the name of Hans Selye discovered that all living tissue undergoes a general adaptation process whereby after infection or stress, the cellular activity increases, forming barriers and strengthening surrounding tissue so that it will be able to handle future stress. Whether scientifically understood at the time or not, the principle was applied to training as far back as mid-500 BC by Milo of Crotona, a farmer who lifted a calf every day while it grew to become a full-grown cow. It is considered the first application of one of our founding exercise principles (see the section "Gradual Progressive Overload").

In the past few years, we have gained more insight into the tiny details of muscle physiology and have begun to combine laboratory animal research with human practical applications. We have found that muscle responds similarly in everyone, male or female, young or old, and that differences in results between persons are likely due to the type of training applied. Initially, much of the debate over size and strength gains focused on genetics; it is now understood that the specific nature of the training protocol is the most important factor.

This new information bodes well for all of you who label yourselves "hard gainers." No matter when you begin your weight training program, you can expect to see remarkable results over time with the right training program.

Train hard, train properly, and you will see favorable results. The key is to decide what results you would like to achieve and then set out on your journey so that your destination matches your goals.

To get the specific results you want, you also need a plan and a commitment to working out. Many infomercials would have you believe that you can see results by working out for as little as a few minutes a couple of times per week, but it is not that easy. No you do not have to become an exercise addict. Neither do you have to make complete life-altering changes. But you do have to make a point of hitting the gym a few times a week for at least 30 minutes. Ideally, though, your workouts will be 60 to 75 minutes, including your warm-up and cool-down. Although you can get results with less, the best way to achieve success is to do it right. There really is no fast track, but there is a smart track that ensures success in the long run.

The amount of exercise needed to produce results is a hotly debated topic. One of the key ingredients in your exercise prescription is figuring out the right amount so that your body can recover, rebuild, and prepare for the next workout.

# WEIGHT TRAINING PRINCIPLES

If you are to derive any real benefits from training, you need to understand the underlying principles of weight training. These principles provide guidance and a foundation for any well-designed training program.

## Frequency, Intensity, Time, and Type (FITT)

FITT is the guiding principle by which all exercise programs are created. The variables of frequency, intensity, time, and type refer to the number of times you exercise, how many times you perform specific exercises, the length of the workout, and which exercises you perform. When developing your exercise program, almost everything you do within the program itself and during your day and week as a whole will have an effect on the outcome of your training program. If you exercise too frequently, you will not make the proper gains and may succumb to overtraining, a physiological term for your body's inability to recover properly. And if you work out too few times, you likely will not see any results from your efforts because your body hasn't been stressed enough to adapt.

On average, the weight training portion of your workout should last no more than one hour, and you should choose 10 to 12 exercises per workout. Training three times a week is ideal; however, any number of times a week is better than no times a week. Although a more advanced lifter may train four or five times a week, it is important to respect your body's ability to recover. Take at least 24 and preferably 48 hours of rest between workouts training the same body areas. As you will see in the exercise chapters, you can use a variety of equipment for resistance, including dumbbells, plate weight barbells, machines, resistance tubing, and even your own body weight.

## Gradual Progressive Overload

Gradual progressive overload (GPO) follows two individual principles: overload and progression. The overload principle states that the body must receive a stimulus greater than it is used to in order to gain any major benefits. That doesn't mean the body will not benefit from using a lesser stimulus; however, greater adaptation takes place when the stress is larger than normal. Overload can be in the form of increasing the resistance (or intensity level), duration (length of time) of activity, frequency of activity, and type of activity, or a combination of any of these variables.

Now wait a moment. Don't just rush off to the gym, load up the bar with a ton of weight, and try to lift it. Remember, your body isn't prepared to handle a lot of weight, especially if you are a beginner. The principle of progression says to start gradually and add a little to each workout. That means either increasing the weight used by a small amount, usually 5 to 10 pounds (2.5 to 5 kg), or trying to perform a few more reps (with perfect form, of course). The most common reason for injury is progressing too fast, so before you make any increase in your workout, be sure that you have truly mastered the previous weight and are really ready to move on. The decision to increase either weight or reps depends on your desired outcome.

## Individuality and Specificity

Okay, so you're ready now. Or are you? Let's say you want to go exercise with your buddy. Is your friend the same age, height, weight, and build as you? If not, then you must realize that there will be some differences in how much weight you use, how you perform the exercises, and the benefits you each receive. This difference is known as individuality.

The principle of individuality simply recognizes that everyone is different and that exercise programs should be designed with these differences in mind. Before you begin to exercise, you need to understand that everyone has different physical attributes, abilities, interests, motivations, and improvement rates. All of these factors should be considered when developing a training routine.

In addition to individualizing your workouts, you need to choose equipment and techniques that will help you achieve the results you want. This is called the specificity principle. Your body will respond and make improvements that are specific to the type of stimulus placed on it. In other words, to see specific results, you must target the muscle you want to develop or the sport-specific skill you want to improve.

The body is an amazing piece of machinery, and it responds to how it is treated. Individual muscles or groups of muscles adapt specifically to the type of training done. For example, if you want to increase the size of your biceps muscle, you should do arm curls. Although this sounds like common sense, it is often not practiced in the weight room. If you walk into the typical weight room, you will see people doing all kinds of crazy things, many of which do not follow the principle of specificity. If you can't see a direct benefit from an exercise, then there probably isn't one.

Although the recommended exercise prescription is one to three sets of 8 to 12 reps of a variety of exercises covering all your muscle groups, specific individual goals need to be considered. If one set program worked for everyone, we would all be doing it and there would be no need for different training programs. In chapter 16 you will find programs for specific goals, but those too may need tweaking to fit your exact needs.

## Adaptation

You have a great chance right now to help yourself for the rest of your life. Because your body will adapt to the weight training you do, you can obtain several benefits. Resistance training offers lifelong benefits. You can expect improvement in muscle strength and endurance, increases in muscle size, stronger bones, and improvement in your overall appearance and feeling of well-being. Lifting weights will even help you burn more fat. Your body will make these specific adaptations in response to your properly progressed weight training routine. Adaptation is also the reason why people gain weight and lose strength and flexibility when they do nothing.

When you weight train, the adaptation your body undergoes is directly due to the application of the FITT principle and the specific nature of how you apply it. This concept is often called SAID (specific adaptation to imposed demand). Your body will improve only in the areas that you try to develop. So if your program does not address all of your body parts at least some time within your workout week, only the parts you train will show results. If you have ever seen guys with large upper bodies walking around on what appear to be popsicle stick legs, you can see that they missed a few exercises, and so their legs don't show any adaptation or improvement.

## Recovery

One of the most important exercise concepts is often the most overlooked and underplanned. Your body will need a break, but only if you work out hard. For those who work out here and there, trying to hit a workout in between several off days, this doesn't apply to you. But for those knocking it out of the park every time, you will need some rest. Your ability to do the next set is a function of how hard you work on the set before and how you want your body to adapt. If you are looking for endurance, you want short breaks, but if you are looking for strength, your rest between sets should be considerably longer.

Beyond the sets is the entire workout. How much time you need to recover is again a function of the intensity you work at and the overall volume. The greater the work, the longer the rest you will need. The 24 to 48 rule is more a generalization as it has been known to take super heavy lifters 96 hours to a full week to recover from an intense training session. The exact amount of rest is still unknown; however, a few symptoms can tell you whether you should have taken a break sooner. The telltale signs that recovery is not working for you are much like those of being sick: weakness, tightness, general uneasiness, increased heart rate, shortness of breath, and inability to focus and function as normal. In other words, if the quality of your workouts is decreasing, you are not recovering.

# 2

# WEIGHT ROOM LANGUAGE AND PROTOCOL

No doubt your first time in a gym may be a bit overwhelming. Even seasoned gym goers get that uncomfortable feeling when something new is introduced. You probably have questions such as "What do I wear?" and "Where do I go?" and you may wonder if people will be staring at you and thinking you look out of place. Chances are good that you will feel like the new student at a school. Don't worry. We have all been there. Most people are not even paying attention if they are serious about their own training. Someone who's staring is either a trainer looking to pull you in as a client or a person wasting time and probably no one you need to worry about. Starting a weight training program at a gym is intimidating and is the number one reason why people don't work out! This chapter arms you with the basics so you understand what to wear, what to say, and most important how to act so that you are not easily identified as a newbie.

Learning the language of the gym can also help you feel more comfortable and allow you to communicate clearly. Much of the terminology used by weightlifters has developed from the anger, frustration, happiness, and success people have experienced in the gym. Some terms are part of the basic language of exercise. Many describe particular techniques or strategies. Others are simply words lifters use to describe how they feel when they lift weights. Learning this language, like any, can be difficult because new words are added daily, exercise names are modified, and the language isn't the same everywhere. But no matter how you say it, as long as you understand the essentials, you will get by fine whether at home in your local gym or when traveling.

## CLOTHING AND ACCESSORIES

The great thing about weight training is that you don't need to rush off to the store to buy new clothes the way you would for some other sports. Except for a few guidelines, pretty much anything goes. Wear loose, comfortable clothing to permit easy movement, allow full range of motion, and increase overall comfort. A good pair of shoes will absorb pressure at the ankles, knees, and lower back during leg work and standing exercises. If you wear jewelry, make sure it cannot get caught in any moving parts of the machines you use, or better yet, just leave it at home. Rings, in particular, can pinch fingers, possibly causing blisters.

A pair of gloves that fit well will prevent the development of calluses. Gloves serve no other functional purpose in weight training. Not wearing gloves will force your hands to toughen up against the bar's knurly surface. So the decision to wear them or not is a matter of personal preference.

Avoid using wrist straps, knee wraps, and belts. These devices tend to prevent strengthening of the wrists, knees, and trunk. When extra support is given to weak joint areas, those areas do not develop the strength they need. Such crutches are needed only when you have an injury; otherwise you will not benefit from their use. True, the initial few workouts will potentially make your wrists and knees sore, but this will also be the time when you strengthen them to withstand further stresses.

Quite interesting and generally unknown is that a belt serves as a wall for the abdominal muscles—not your back muscles—to press against. This raises the pressure in your trunk and forces your lower back to stabilize. Although weak abdominals is the reason most often cited for using belts, the longer you use a belt, the longer it will take to strengthen your back and abdominals. Having said that, it is advisable to use a belt when lifting very heavy weights to ensure that you have enough support, but for routines using light to moderate weights, a belt is not necessary.

Wearing the right clothes and shoes will get you started on the right track, and the rest of this chapter will finish preparing you for other characteristics of gym culture. However, don't forget that before you hoist that first barbell, you will need to prepare your body for action. In chapter 4, you will learn about warming up, cooling down, and stretching. All three elements are vital to a good exercise program.

# GYM ETIQUETTE

Understanding the unwritten rules of the gym will help you know what to do and what not to do and will make you a favorite of the staff and other gym members. Plus, you will feel more comfortable when you begin training because you will reduce the number of unfriendly interactions. The following rules will help you navigate the gym floor as if you've been lifting for years.

- **Avoid walking in front of anyone who is completing a set.** No matter how tempting it may be, never do this. It is very distracting to the person lifting. Walk behind the person, or wait until the set is over. Yes, the person lifting may be standing right in front of the rack of weights (and he shouldn't be standing there—see the next rule), but you, being the well-mannered gym patron that you are, will wait your turn.

- **Provide plenty of space.** You are not the only person in the gym. If you are standing in front of the entire dumbbell rack, step back, move to the side, or take your dumbbells to another area. Let others have access to the equipment. Don't crowd an area, either. Make sure to give people a little extra personal space, both for safety and for comfort.

- **Look before you leap.** As this old saying goes, you need to think about your next move. Remember, safety is first and foremost. Before you pick up a bar and start walking, take a look around. Almost all gym accidents happen because people just don't pay attention to their surroundings.

- **Clean up the equipment.** C'mon, nobody else wants your germs or needs to bathe in your sweat. Do your part by keeping your bench clean. Most gyms offer a towel and have cleaners available if you make a mess, but if not, at least bring your own towel.

- **Share and be polite.** "Can I jump in?" is a common question heard in gyms. If you can't let someone else use the equipment in between your sets, chances are you are not lifting hard enough. You need a rest, they need to lift; this seems like an obvious compromise.

- **Spot rather than stare.** It is easy to stand around and watch someone squirming about on a bench. Don't wonder what is going on, either help or move on. Yes, some people do some strange things. Some are correct, and some are not, but keep in mind what comes around, goes around. You wouldn't want to be the freak show everyone else was looking at, would you?

- **Rack your weights.** If everyone did this, the gym would be clean and you wouldn't spend 10 minutes looking for another 5-pound (2.5 kg) plate. Treat a gym like your own home; picking up after yourself makes it better for the next person. And for those of you who lift super heavy, take the time to unload the leg press. Besides, if you are that strong, it should be a piece of cake for you.

# BASIC WEIGHT PROGRAM LANGUAGE

To get the most out of your workout, you need to understand the basic language of lifting weights. Like any activity, knowing the basic terminology will help you plan your workout better and reach your goals sooner.

## Reps and Sets

The repetition—the execution of a movement in both directions—is the foundation for improvement and the basis for each exercise. A single repetition (*rep* for short) consists of an eccentric contraction (the negative portion of a movement in most cases) in which the muscle lengthens and a concentric contraction (the positive portion of the movement) in which the muscle shortens. For example, with a simple dumbbell curl for the biceps, flexing your arm while pulling the weight up toward your shoulder from your waist is the concentric action, while lowering the weight back down (opening up your arm) is the eccentric action.

Performing repetitions in succession without a break between them is considered a *set* of repetitions. However, what truly defines a set is the break taken between each grouping of consecutive repetitions. A set may be prolonged with a momentary pause that may last even a few seconds to catch your breath, helping you get a few more reps, but the full set is the point when the weight is finally put down. That break, or rest period, indicates the set has ended. Rep and set notation is written as *X sets of Y reps*. For example, three of 10 means three sets of 10 repetitions.

Before you begin to exercise, however, you need to understand that the manner in which you perform reps will have an impact on how your muscle develops. Probably the single most important thing to remember is that every rep needs to be done properly. For success, you must strive to execute the perfect rep on each and every attempt. This prevents you from developing bad lifting habits, reduces your chances of injury, and improves your chances of developing quality musculature. This most basic concept will come back to haunt you if you are not careful. Once you have perfected your technique, it is important to understand how a simple change in how much or how often you lift can make a huge difference in your rate of achieving your goals.

## Load and Resistance

*Load* and *resistance* are the scientific terms to describe an externally applied force that the body must overcome. The term *weights* has been used as the catchall term for all resistance and is often confused since there are so many ways to create resistance to challenge the body. Thus the term *resistance training* is more accurate than weight training in that it refers to any and all external ways of creating a load for the body to lift. The term *load* itself is more accurate as it refers directly to the work required to perform a task. Furthermore, the word *lifting* as part of *weightlifting* is also a bit of a misnomer in that, unless you are referring specifically to an external weight that moves against gravity, not all exercises require lifting. Some are pushes, and some are pulls. If this all sounds a bit complicated, don't worry; in the exercise chapters you will see how many different ways an external load can be applied. Many programs in today's training routines use medicine balls, resistance tubing, and your own body weight in addition to the plate-loaded barbells, dumbbells, and fancy resistance machines.

## Rest

We all know what rest is, so to include it in this list of terms may seem unnecessary. However, rest is essential for building an effective program, determining the amount of resistance you need, and seeing your hard work pay off through proper recovery. Chapter 15 further discusses the importance of rest, but for now, know that when you need to rest helps determine if you're working at the proper intensity. If you don't need a rest between your three sets of 12-rep exercises, then you are not working hard enough.

Rest is crucial between sets for recovery to go on to the next set, and simply by manipulating a few seconds here and there, you can completely change your workout.

## Volume

Another important concept is how much work you are going to do per set, per exercise, and per workout. The total amount of work you perform can actually be measured, and it is kind of neat to see how much you really lift. It is not uncommon for the average male to lift the equivalent of the amount of furniture in an entire house during a workout! You can calculate volume using the following equation:

$$\text{weight} \times \text{reps} \times \text{sets} = \text{volume}$$

You simply multiply the weight lifted by the number of reps by the number of sets. For example, someone who uses 100 pounds (45 kg) for a bench press exercise for three sets of 10 reps lifts 3,000 pounds (1,350 kg) of weight (100 × 10 × 3). Volume is a relative piece of information, though. Coaches use total volume for developing specific programs as well as helping with tapering (the gradual reduction of total volume in a workout to help with recovery) for competition. But for the average person, volume is a cool number that gives you an idea of how much total work you did in a training session. Since volume really depends on the person and the type of exercise and rest periods that are chosen, it is a difficult tool to use at first. In general, the greater the volume in a particular program, the faster you will see results, assuming your body can recover effectively. If your body cannot recover, then your volume is too high.

# LIFTING AND TRAINING TERMINOLOGY

When you walk in to a gym or fitness facility for the first time, you should be familiar with some general terms, as no doubt an aggressive salesperson or trainer will tackle you with terms that will make you feel as if you missed a whole developmental stage of your life. Knowing what you are doing is half the battle. Understanding some general lifting and training terminology will help you understand what people are saying, will help you feel more comfortable when working out, and of course, will prevent you from looking as if you have never been in a gym.

- **Abduction** refers to moving a limb away from the midline of the body. For example, if your arm is down at your side and you move it out and up to shoulder height (so your armpit makes a 90-degree angle), your arm is now abducted.

- **Adduction** refers to moving a limb toward the midline of the body. For example, if your arm is up at shoulder height (your armpit makes a

90-degree angle) in the abducted position and you bring it back down toward your side, you are adducting it.

- **Alternative resistance devices** are any type of external way to produce resistance that is unconventional from that of a machine or free weights, such as specialized tubing, medicine balls, stability balls, and other objects.

- **Concentration exercises** are specific single-joint exercises that isolate a particular muscle. Most commonly, the biceps, triceps, hamstrings, and quadriceps have variations of their normal movements that call for specific isolation.

- **Extension** is the act of increasing the joint angle. For example, if you are sitting and you lift a leg straight out in front, you are extending the knee.

- **Flexion** is the opposite of extension. This is a confusing term because we use the word *flex* to describe "making a muscle," as in flexing the biceps. The anatomical term and gym jargon are slightly different. Anatomically, flexion is decreasing the joint angle. The gym term probably arose from the fact that you flex your arm (make the joint angle smaller) to make your biceps bulge (flex the muscle).

- **Group training** is any training session that has more than one participant. Gone are the days of the original aerobics classes. Today's classes incorporate tubing, balls, dumbbells, bicycles, and other devices. Also, personal training has developed from the standard one-on-one session to small groups (similar to that of an athletic program at a high school or college) to ease individual budgets while increasing trainer's hourly rate.

- **Free weight** is the catchall term for anything that is not a machine. Dumbbells, barbells, and plates are free weights. Generally, free weight plates are added to bars to increase the total resistance, but some machines also allow for additional weight to be added. Don't let the name fool you, though; they are certainly not free when it comes to the price. Although inexpensive plates and bars are available at a variety of sporting goods stores, high-quality equipment is expensive. In fact, rubber-coated special plates and those used by Olympic and high-level athletes can cost more than $5 per pound (per .5 kg). The bars themselves can run more than $1,200 each.

- **Isolateral** is a fancy term that means each arm or leg moves individually. *Iso* stands for isolation, and *lateral* refers to either side.

- **Locking out** refers to completing the entire repetition and finishing with the joint or joints fully extended. Although some people are against locking out, if done gently, you increase your total range of motion, increasing the overall length and shape of your muscle. You should never "snap" into place, but a soft lock is definitely recommended.

- **Machines** are anything that either has preloaded weight or can add external weight while maintaining a specific line of movement for control and stabilization. Machines that move in a set path provide greater stabilization and focus more on isolating specific muscles. Some companies believe that this specific line is too strict and have created machines that work along multiple paths, forcing other muscles to get involved as well as creating greater variation for the lifter. The multiple paths approach attempts to make a machine more like a free weight. Some machines work well this way while others do not, making the machine more cumbersome and the movement more difficult to perform. Since both isolation of muscle and incorporating multiple muscles are desired, a training program should use both fixed machines and those with adjustable settings. Machines that use pulleys and cables allow for greater range of motion, which in turn allows the lifter to create many different exercises using the same machine. However, with a cable you need better technique and control; thus the true beginner should focus on machines with a set path of motion.

- **Multijoint (or compound) exercises** involve more than one joint and are oriented more toward sport and real-life movement since they are not isolated. For example, a lat pull-down involves the same muscles of the elbow as the dumbbell curl as well as the muscles that cross the shoulder joint. Multijoint exercises are the preferred choice when time is limited or when looking for a movement-based approach rather than isolation.

- **Personal trainer**, **facility manager**, **group fitness manager**, and **floor staff** are all fancy terms given to gym staff members. True personal trainers have certifications or college-level education in exercise science and training. They can be a great source of information when you are looking for help, a few ideas, or full-scale training services to push yourself beyond your own means. However, be careful when joining large-chain gyms that have all kinds of fees and offer many services in an expensive building with high-end equipment. Many of the staff are merely pawns of the sales game looking to sell you anything they can. Although this is not true of all facilities, be wary, be armed, and understand what you are getting into. Take your time, and pick a training center where you feel most comfortable.

- **Plate-loading machines** are ones where you have to put the weight on yourself. Generally, there will be a bar or pole to place plates on, and you select your load by increasing the number of plates you add.

- **Single-joint (or isolation) exercises** focus on the muscles of a single joint. A dumbbell curl involving the muscles surrounding the single elbow joint is the best example. These exercises are best for working specific hard-to-grow muscles or to specifically isolate a particular muscle.

- **21s** are just one of many ways to add variety to your training routine. The number refers to the total number of reps. Specifically, you perform 7 reps of half of the movement, 7 of the other half of the movement, and

7 of the complete movement one after another. This approach is generally used when doing arm curls but can be used for any part of the body.

• **Weight stack**, **adjustable**, and **pin-loading machines** are common machines that have a preset weight stack, and you select the actual load you are looking to lift. The pin is a tool that helps you select the appropriate weight by placing it in the stack at the weight level you desire; it is easily adjustable if the weight is too light or too heavy.

# GYM JARGON

Once you are a regular at the gym, you may hear many words that sound as if they are related to training, but the exact meaning may be unclear if you're new to weight training. Welcome to gym jargon, a language started mostly by pumped-up behemoth bodybuilders and powerlifters that is now common in most gyms. Like any language, at first it seems awkward, but many of the terms are descriptive, and since the true science behind weight training came long after people started doing it, little thought went into the creation of new words. The list of terms that follows will give you a good introduction to the jargon you're likely to hear in the gym. When you have a clear understanding of gym jargon, you should have no trouble standing up to the 300-pound, 6-foot-5 (135 kg, 195 cm) monster and asking for a spot or politely telling him to rack his weights. Then flex your tiny pistols and get back to work on making the perfect peak.

• *Arnold* is the man who fashioned the art of building muscle and brought it to the popularity it is today. He stands alone as the only person in the world of muscle who needs no last name—besides it is hard to spell. If you're still not sure who this is, you may know him better as Governor Schwarzenegger.

• *Cannons* (also known as *guns*, *wings*, *bazookas*, and *jacks*) describe the upper arms. Generally, the larger the arm circumference, the greater the size of your gun. *Wings* means that the size of your arms is birdlike. Why that has anything to do with lifting, I'm not sure. Similarly, the origin of the term *jacks* is unclear, but it could be from the fact that a jack is used to lift something, and you lift with your arms. Gym jargon can be confusing, even irrational at times, but you will end up using these terms in time—everyone does.

• *Cheat reps* are a way to complete a repetition without help from a spotter but with help from other muscles. Usually, a cheat is in the form of a bounce or momentum used to get over the sticking point. These can be ugly and very dangerous to both the lifter and those around him. Notice I said *him*; women rarely use cheat reps, preferring to focus more on precision.

• *Crush it* is used as hyperbole to create aggression and inspiration to make one lift harder and stronger. It means to crush the set or rep, not the weight itself (that would be nearly impossible). You may hear a training partner, coach, or spotter yell, "Crush it!"

- *Cut* (and *chiseled*, *shredded*, *sliced*, and *diced*) refers to a person's overall percentage of body fat. Those with superior skills at dieting and perfectly trimming their fat to make their muscles pop are considered to be among the very few that receive these super terms. In the bodybuilding world, you generally need to have a body fat of less than 6 percent if you truly want to be considered chiseled. In fact since this is such a difficult level to achieve (and certainly not something I suggest you attempt), we further use terms such as "cut like glass"—something difficult to do and very precise. Those lean enough are considered to have paper-thin skin, so nearly every vein in the body is visible. What this really means is that their subcutaneous fat is almost nonexistent.

- *Cuts*, *lines*, and *hardness* are also terms for being lean but generally refer to the specific quality of a muscle and its shape. You may have nice lines or hardness in one area but are still not shredded enough to be considered super lean.

- *Help* is a word you seldom like to hear in a gym since it means you may be in trouble. It is especially bad to hear when you are pinned underneath a bar during a heavy lift. It is also a way to describe forced reps, generally to refer to a set that was completed with a little extra influence from the spotter. Keep in mind that forced reps, a method of training to get an extra couple reps in your set, is a form of help. Requiring a spotter to provide a little extra help to complete the set is a good thing. Requiring a group of people or a forklift to lift the entire pile of weight off you is not.

- *It's all you* is a good way to tell your training partner that he is lifting all the weight himself, and you are there only if a true spot is needed. Although in some cases this acts as a nice motivator, often it results in the spotters getting much bigger forearms and trapezius muscles as they tend to be lifting quite a bit more than needed, making it all them! A spot is designed to help a lifter continue and complete a set not so the spotter gets a workout. It is common to see many guys trying to lift very heavy weight in the gym, while often their partners are doing quite a bit of the work. If this is the case, you are lifting too much weight. In other words, if your training partner is developing pulling muscles (such as traps when lifting upward) faster than you are developing your push muscles (as in a bench press), then you need to cut back on the weight.

- *Master Blaster* is the name given to pioneer fitness magazine legend Joe Weider, who began writing and training before most of you were even born. The term is often given to others to describe their talent as the king of a domain.

- *Peak* usually refers to the fully flexed biceps muscle poking out of your shirt like the apex of a mountain. It can be used to describe other muscles or the moment in your workout where you reached your maximal weight or effort.

- *Pins* (along with *wheels*, *poles*, and *dogs*) is used to describe the legs. *Pins* may be large, as when referring to the legs as bowling pins, which are more round at the bottom, or small, as when referring to something like the thinness of a safety pin. Again, if you are confused, so are the people who started using these terms. *Wheels* is used to describe the legs as a whole since like a car's wheels, they are the parts that roll you along. The term is often used to describe the training day, as in "I'm training wheels today." If your legs are small in relation to the rest of your body, they may be referred to as *toothpicks*, *chopsticks*, *poles*, *pins*, or anything small and thin. Generally if your legs are large, you may be given the name Quadzilla. People usually use the word *dogs* in a sentence referring to a hard-core leg pump: "My dogs are barking."

- *Pump* refers to increasing blood flow to the muscles, which makes them bulge and, when lean enough, may bring out veins. It is typically used when a person believes she has gotten a really good workout. Men like to get a good pump, and that is obvious, but women do as well if they want their arms or legs to look shapely when wearing a sleeveless top or a skirt.

- *Squeeze* and *flex* are terms used to create maximal tension in the muscle to force it to bulge as much as possible. Bodybuilders will squeeze at the fully flexed position to enhance the feel and get a better pump.

- *Sticking point* is the point in an exercise where your leverage is at its worst possible point. Typically it is midway through a lift but varies depending on many factors. You always have a sticking point because of the anatomical makeup of your body and the biomechanical factors that dictate movement. When the weight is light enough, you will not notice the sticking point; but as the weight increases, it will be evident, and you will want to do what you can to overcome it.

- *Sweep* is the roundness that a large outer thigh makes sweeping from the hip down to the knee. Although you want a defined leg, when not flexing, it should be lean and rounded.

- *Taper* and *V* describe the shape of the upper body as it narrows from the shoulders to the waist. If you have those pesky love handles, it is unlikely that you will be considered to have this shape. Although the taper or V shape is usually used to describe men's torsos, it also forms the top portion of the hourglass figure often used when describing women.

- *Washboard*, *cubes in the tray*, and *six pack* specifically refer to the abdominal region and being able to see the individual parts of the entire front abdominal muscle. Interestingly, there are eight parts of this abdominal muscle (known as the rectus abdominis), but since most people never get that lean and a six pack is well known, the term *eight pack* never made it except to describe a pack of batteries or hot dog buns.

# 3

# TYPES OF RESISTANCE TRAINING

Deciding which exercises to perform in a workout can be a tricky task. Chapters 5 through 14 present many of the most common exercises for various parts of the body, and in chapter 15, you will select how to put your program together and decide which body parts, specific muscles, or movement patterns to focus on. Surprisingly, those decisions may be easier than deciding what method of resistance training you will use to perform the exercises you select. Since there are many ways to perform the same exercise, the choice is truly yours because no one method is better than another.

The principle of individuality as described in chapter 1 says that no two persons are the same, and thus you will find that some exercises feel and work better for you than others. In some cases, you will find an exercise uncomfortable or just not enjoyable. Fortunately, since there are so many ways to get the job done, there is an option that will work for you.

The philosophies about how to approach your workout are as diverse as the exercise selection. By learning the different resistance methods, you create more options when it comes to building your program. One specific exercise may be performed using several forms of resistance, creating many new exercises of which one should work for you. Additionally, when you tie in the principles in chapter 1 with methods and types of exercise combinations, you can achieve the look you want and the perfect workout for you. So whether you work out at home, in your office, or in the gym, there is definitely a solution to help you achieve your goals. This chapter helps you navigate the waters of the weight room and choose the right exercises.

## TOOLS

Every occupation or sport has its tools necessary for performance. The world of weight training also has its shed of handyman resources. And like any great craft, the larger your shed and the fuller it is, the more options you have. But before you go filling your toolbox with unnecessary equipment, it is wise to understand what you really need, especially if you are a beginner. Unfortunately, there are many equipment manufacturers with gimmicky devices that claim they can do it all for you. Most of these items end up being a clothes

# Comparing Different Types of Resistance

| Type of resistance | Pros | Cons |
|---|---|---|
| Barbell free weight | Develops balance<br>Works stabilizer muscles<br>Presents a challenge for most | Requires a partner<br>Requires skill or technique that may take a long time to learn<br>Does not isolate muscles |
| Dumbbell free weight | Is excellent for rehab<br>Allows for working out alone<br>Allows for movement in any direction<br>Simulates just about any movement | Requires skill<br>May cause lost emphasis of exercise in trying to balance the weight and move evenly |
| Isolateral machine | Allows for weaker arm or leg to be developed individually<br>Is excellent for rehab<br>Isolates muscles<br>Allows for working out alone | Does not allow for good development of stabilizer muscles |
| Bilateral machine | Is excellent for rehab<br>Isolates muscles<br>Allows for working out alone | Does not allow for good development of stabilizer muscles<br>May not provide enough of a challenge for some |
| Cable-pulley machine | Is excellent for rehab<br>Allows for working out alone<br>Allows for movement in any direction<br>Simulates just about any movement | Requires stabilization, increased technical skill, and strong core musculature |
| Isokinetic machine | Causes muscles to produce maximal force throughout the entire range of motion at a specific controlled velocity | Is very expensive and highly impractical |
| Body weight | Develops the muscle completely along the entire strength curve<br>Is an excellent additional way to help with endurance training | May not provide enough resistance<br>May provide too much resistance in certain movements |
| Manual resistance | Develops the muscle completely along the entire strength curve<br>Can be applied to any of the above or by itself<br>Is probably the best method for training | Requires two people<br>Does not allow for easy measurement of strength gains<br>Does not provide a visual of the weight<br>Requires knowledge of how to properly apply the resistance |
| Resistance tubing and bands | Are excellent for rehab<br>Allow for working out alone<br>Allow for movement in any plane<br>Simulate just about any movement<br>Are excellent for explosive lifting | Do not allow for easy measurement of strength gains<br>May not provide enough resistance<br>Change strength curve over stretch (starts out easier, gets tougher)<br>Do not provide a visual of the weight |
| Medicine ball | Adds variety<br>Is excellent for increasing range of motion<br>Is excellent for core muscle development and explosive weight training | Is hard to control<br>Does not allow for easy measurement of strength gains<br>Does not isolate muscles |
| Kettlebell | Is excellent for rehab<br>Allows for working out alone<br>Allows for movement in any direction<br>Simulates just about any movement | Requires skill<br>May cause lost emphasis of exercise in trying to balance the weight and move evenly |

hanger or find a permanent home under your bed. Fortunately, all you need is your body, perhaps a little resistance tubing or a few dumbbells, and if you want, a gym membership.

With so many choices, it is often difficult to decide what to do each time you hit the gym, but that in itself is what makes your program both interesting and effective. In some cases your choice of equipment is dictated by the gym itself or your financial position, but most important is how you choose to exercise, not what you exercise with. High-end machines, souped-up treadmills and bikes, and super-clean lockers do not guarantee better results, although the latter does make your experience more enjoyable. Instead, what is most important is knowing what you want to achieve in your training program. In fact, your most powerful tool is your mind. If you know why you are choosing a particular exercise, if you perform the movement properly, and if you believe in your actions, good results are inevitable. This means that despite the shortcomings of your home gym or the plethora of machines at your fitness club, you have to choose which tool is right for the job, and if there isn't one, make one that is. If a simple hammer were all that is needed to drive in a nail, why are there so many different kinds?

## Free Weights

Free weights consist of barbells (see figure 3.1), which are long bars, and dumbbells, which are shorter barbells that are usually intended for use with one hand. Barbells and dumbbells may have fixed or adjustable weights. Many gyms have several kinds of barbells, including cambered bars, which

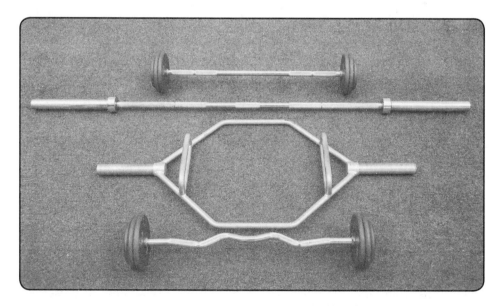

**Figure 3.1** Common types of barbells include a straight bar, full bar, trap bar, and cambered bar.

are bent in the middle to allow for a different hand grip, and trap bars, which are specifically designed for floor-to-waist lifts (figure 3.1). Trap bars center the weight over your line of pull instead of out in front. They have a diamond shape in the middle that the lifter stands in, allowing for a neutral grip (palms in toward your sides) and for the bar to travel straight up and down. Specially shaped bars that fit on the ends of pulley machines and allow for different grips are also available. A full-length gym barbell weighs about 45 pounds (20 kg). Shorter barbells generally weigh about 20 pounds (9 kg).

In general, bars are knurled (the k is silent), meaning they are textured rather than smooth to allow for better grip. Olympic-style bars have a deep, smooth groove that can help you line your hands up properly. Most Olympic bars have two areas of deep knurling, roughly 32 inches (81 cm) apart from each other in the middle of the bar. These act as perfect guides for spacing your hands differently. The decision of where to place your hands is based on the goal of the exercise, but in general, you want to take a slightly wider than shoulder-width grip, which for many has their pinkies touching the deep knurl.

Standard non-Olympic-style free bars have $1\frac{1}{8}$-inch (3 cm) diameter ends on which weight plates fit. Olympic free weight bars have sleeves that create a larger 2-inch (5 cm) diameter end for Olympic plates to fit on. The sleeves are designed to allow the weight to spin so that as you move the weight through an arc motion, you create less stress against your wrist. With both types of free bars, the plates that are added need to be held on with collars so the plates don't slide off if you become slightly off balance. The $1\frac{1}{8}$-inch collars come standard, but Olympic bar collars come in a variety of styles. The most common gym style is the simple lightweight clip-on type that fits on the end of the bar by squeezing the ends of the collar clip together (see figure 3.2). Competition-style collars are heavy duty to hold back very heavy weights, and each weighs 5 pounds (2.5 kg) on its own. Regardless of the type, collars are a must. Many gym accidents have occurred as a result of the weights sliding off one side of a bar. Both standard and Olympic plates range from 1.25 pounds (.5 kg) to 100 pounds (45 kg). In international competition and Olympic lifting, plates are measured in kilograms and range from .5 kilograms to 25 kilograms. Plates come in a variety of shapes, with some having handles, rubber coating, or specific colors.

Unlike bars with adjustable weights, fixed barbells are locked in place and do not allow the weights to spin, do not need collars, and usually range from 10 pounds (5 kg) to more than 150 pounds (70 kg). Fixed dumbbells also come in a variety of shapes and can range from 1 pound (.5 kg) to more than 200 pounds (90 kg) each.

Fixed and adjustable benches and racks complement free weights, improving safety and increasing the variety of exercises that can be performed. Fixed benches for the bench press and incline bench press are standard in most training facilities, as are flat and adjustable utility benches that can be moved around the room. Most benches are 16 to 18 inches (40-45 cm) high, which fits most people, but if you are shorter or taller you may find some benches or their positions uncomfortable. If you are uncomfortable, chances are you

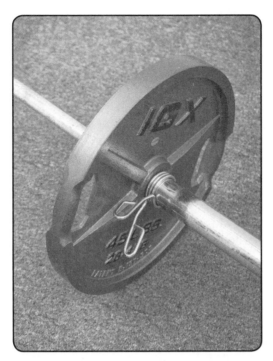

**Figure 3.2** Many gyms use a simple clip-on type collar clip to hold weight plates in place.

will not benefit from the exercise. You have two choices: Find a way to fit, or choose a different exercise. Shorter persons can place large 45-pound plates (or any thick plate) under their feet, giving them that little extra height. Taller people, unfortunately, may just need to find a different exercise.

A power rack completes the free weight equipment list and is designed for doing squats and other heavy-duty lifts. Since the racks come with built-in supports and safety stops, they can be useful for many other lifts by simply pulling up an adjustable bench.

The advantages of free weight lifting are that it provides considerable challenge and develops balance and coordination, making this one of the best choices for overall strength development. Free weights generally offer more exercises and can increase range of motion. Additionally, exercises using dumbbells work arms independently so that essential balance skills can be developed. The disadvantages of free weight exercises are that several require a spotter to assist, and if you are a beginner, the added balance challenge may initially be too great to develop proper lifting technique.

## Weight Machines

The past 15 years have seen an explosion in the number of weight machine manufacturers around the world, and equipment manufacturers have begun creating a wide array of machines that are very different from the straight-motion machines developed in the late 1960s and early 1970s. Although old-school machines did work well, their limited adaptability in both function (how the exercise is performed) and fit (who can use the machine) meant that not everybody could use them in their programs. Now because of the variety available, it is almost impossible to find an argument against machines.

Machines have become very popular in fitness clubs because they are safe and require little instruction, allowing the ratio of lifters to supervisors to be quite high. Machines are designed to help with body position, technique, and stabilization as they follow a specific movement path. Most are designed for bilateral movement in that both limbs, either your arms or legs, move together simultaneously. Most machines are plate loaded or stack loaded. Plate-loaded machines use the same weight plates as free weight bars, while stack-loaded machines come with a complete set of weights built in. Generally, plate-loaded machines allow smaller weight increments as well as heavier loads than most stack machines but offer similar forms of resistance.

Some machines use pulleys, cam systems, and various cables, while others just pivot or rotate against the load. Machines are very good at isolating muscle groups by providing a strict line of pull, making specific muscle building much easier. But now, many machines offer a cabling system that allows for a free range of motion, and some require you to stand and activate your core musculature. Isolateral machines use independent limb systems that simulate dumbbell movements, allowing you to work one leg or one arm at a time. Fixed-line machines have the advantage of not needing a spotter, while standing pulley machines offer the independence of free range of motion.

In a clinical setting, where rehabilitation takes place, you will find a variety of very specialized machines that are designed to measure and control for speed, force production, balance, and other physical characteristics. In particular, isokinetic machines, which control speed of movement—allowing for maximal force production along the entire movement path—are used almost exclusively for research testing and specific weakness. Although these machines provide the most accurate way to address muscle function, their cost and complexity make them unrealistic for use in a gym setting.

A popular plate-loading device is the Smith machine. Essentially, it is similar to a barbell used in a rack except that the barbell is fixed within the confines of the machine. The full-size barbell tracks straight up and down. This specially designed machine allows you to perform more difficult free weight barbell exercises, such as the squat and lunge (seen in chapters 11 and 12), while helping control the weight by providing a set path to help with balance. There have been several variations of the Smith machine since its original design, making it even more adaptable and allowing for even more exercises to be performed. The advantage is that it works like a barbell with the safety and control of a machine.

## Body Weight and Manual Resistance

A long time ago, pull-ups, sit-ups, and push-ups were considered strengthening exercises and were and still are commonly used by the military and law enforcement. For some reason, probably the invention of really cool weightlifting equipment, we have forgotten that our own body weight is often enough resistance to force us to struggle.

If you can do only a few push-ups, it would seem logical that push-ups themselves may be a good choice for upper body strengthening. If you cannot do a single push-up, then a modified version (from your knees) may work well and eventually help you do a regular one. If you are training at home, your body plus possibly a dumbbell or some resistance tubing may be all the resistance you need to make a challenging program. And for a gym-based program, a set of body-weight squats may be the perfect extra endurance kicker to follow a nice set of barbell squats.

Take it one step further and use your strength and body weight to provide resistance for someone else, and you are now doing something called manual resistance. Two people working together can make an excellent team provided they both understand how to help one another. When performing manual resistance training, one person is the spotter and provides the resistance while the other person does the lifting. The person providing resistance can use his own body weight as leverage and needs to provide just enough to make it challenging while also keeping the exercise moving along properly. Manual resistance is basically the opposite of spotting in that you want to push or pull to create resistance opposite to the direction of the movement. The addition of manual resistance to regular exercises allows you to add a little extra challenge. Both body-weight training and manual resistance have been used for decades and should not be overlooked, especially for beginners.

## Alternative Forms of Resistance Training

Over the past several years, the number of alternative forms of resistance training has grown significantly and includes a wide variety of equipment. New types of resistance equipment are being created all the time. As a result, describing every possibility here would be impossible. When determining whether to use any new types of equipment, the most important considerations are safety and effectiveness. If the equipment meets both of these standards and you are interested in adding it to your exercise routine, then go for it. Alternative forms of resistance training equipment that have become popular and that you may encounter at the gym include resistance tubing and bands, medicine balls, and kettlebells.

### Resistance Tubing and Bands

Resistance tubing is inexpensive and can be used anywhere, which makes it a clear choice for home-based training and fieldwork. For the most part, tubing with handles at each end works best (see figure 3.3). This is readily

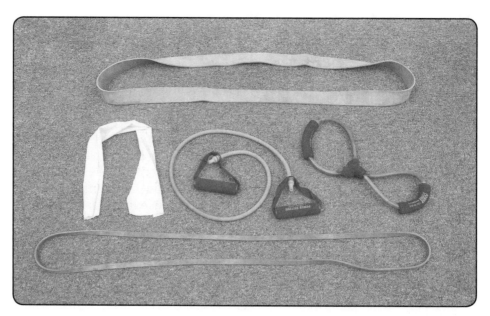

**Figure 3.3**   Various type of resistance tubing and bands are available.

available at local stores or online, and you will need little modification to make exercises beneficial. You may also consider tubing with no handles (you can remove one or both), which may make it easier to tie one end off but more difficult to hold.

With a little creative thinking, you can hook tubing around a post or combine it with a broomstick to simulate almost every free weight exercise found in your gym. Additionally, since tubing comes in a variety of sizes and resistance, this equipment can be modified for just about any movement and to fit any person. It is superior for standing movements, core rotational exercises, and explosive movements and can be found in just about every gym or strength room across the country. The only drawbacks of this method are that it is difficult to track strength gains and heavy lifters may find that there is not enough resistance.

Giant elastic bands (figure 3.3) have also found a place in training programs both as a stand-alone training tool and as additive resistance to normal barbell routines to increase resistance as well as deliver resistance in a different plane. These larger bands create considerably more resistance and may be more appropriate for stronger people or those looking for a greater challenge. As a stand-alone, the bands function similarly to tubing, although you will have to get a little more creative to fix them securely.

## Medicine Balls

Using weighted objects for training dates back to the early 1900s; however, more recently, the use of medicine balls (often referred to as *med balls*) has gained in popularity both in athletics and in health clubs. Med balls are

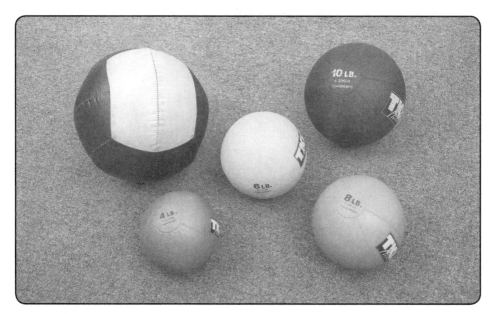

**Figure 3.4** Med balls come in a variety of sizes.

typically made of hard rubber or leather and come in a variety of sizes (see figure 3.4), from 2 pounds (1 kg) up to as much as 30 pounds (15 kg). They have become a great training tool for large groups or those working out at home or with kids.

Above all, medicine balls add variety to the same old routines. Depending on how the medicine ball is applied to the conditioning program, it can serve many purposes. It can be used to develop flexibility and emphasize stretching, muscular endurance, strength, or power. As a pure strength builder, medicine balls are not heavy enough for most people to produce an overload inside the 5 to 8 rep range, but for power, where speed of execution is the goal, medicine balls present a very realistic challenge. Although power training sounds more athletic, for those looking for more lifelike movement patterns, using med balls explosively improves overall fitness, coordination, balance, and control. Another advantage is that med ball training can be done alone or with a partner, and although it is hard to measure gains (similar to tubing), the challenge of controlling the ball improves core strength and stability and adds a lot of variety to your normally dull routine. Since med balls are portable, they can be used anywhere and from any position (standing, sitting, or lying).

## Kettlebells

Another extremely popular alternative training tool that has recently gained much attention is kettlebells (see figure 3.5). They are similar to dumbbells except are solid in form, with a thick handle attached to a solid ball. Kettlebells can be used the same way as dumbbells for regular strength exercises

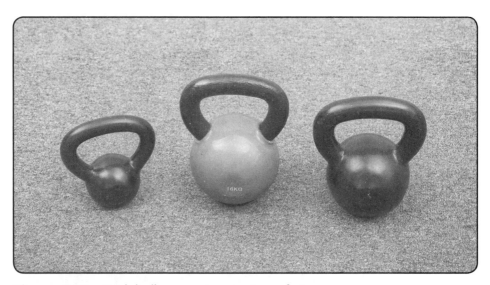

**Figure 3.5**  Kettlebells come in a variety of sizes.

such as curls or presses. They can also be used for more explosive exercises such as cleans and snatches. Kettlebells are not new. In fact, they are one of the older training tools that we have stolen from ancient Roman times. Kettlebells made their mark in the late 1800s, then dropped off the map for nearly 100 years before being brought back in the late 1990s and becoming iconic for some training advocates.

The shape of kettlebells adds variety to normal dumbbell exercises. One factor that differentiates kettlebells from dumbbells is their handle thickness and location relative to the weight, making grip strength and control an additional challenge that you need to get used to before increasing weight and progressing moves. Since a kettlebell's center of gravity is not in the handle (unlike a dumbbell's), the weight is more difficult to control, making forearm and shoulder rotator cuff muscles work harder than if using a similarly weighted dumbbell. Thinner grip and small lightweight kettlebells are available, but using those defeats this unique training advantage of kettlebells. To properly use a kettlebell, you should try to prevent it from falling into your hand. In other words, you should keep the bell up and solid rather than let it flop around. If you allow kettlebells to be loose in your hands, they will smack into your wrists frequently, which could be painful.

Although kettlebells have seen a resurgence, they are merely another tool in your shed. Don't forgo your mainstay exercises to use the kettlebell more. Enthusiasts will have you believe that kettlebells are very different from dumbbells; although they do offer some advantages, kettlebells and dumbbells can be used interchangeably for most exercises. As a training tool, they certainly add variety, but because they come only in fixed weights, they make true progressive resistance training difficult to achieve if you use them exclusively.

## INDEPENDENT ARM MOVEMENT

An easy and productive way to add variety to your workout is to use dumbbells, kettlebells, or tubing. Unlike weight machines, these methods can be used anywhere. They are available in nearly every gym and can even be used in your home. The movements for doing the exercises should be the same as they would be with barbells or weight machines, but dumbbells, kettlebells, and tubing allow each arm to freely move in its own path. This means two things. First, you must use good technique to keep the movement following the proper path. Second, you can alter your arm position so that the movement will be more comfortable. For example, in the bench press, your palms could be turned toward each other instead of facing in the same direction if that is an easier grip for you. Remember, when you use alternative methods, the stabilization normally provided by the weight machine or barbell must be provided by you. Decrease the weight and get control of the dumbbells before you try the tricky stuff.

# TECHNIQUE

Using proper lifting technique is very important. Chapters 5 through 14 explain the proper technique for exercises, but we need to discuss the execution of a rep itself. Every rep needs to be perfect. A properly executed rep consists of moving the weight through a joint's entire range of motion (unless you are injured). A joint's range of motion is the distance the joint can move before bone contacts bone or muscle contacts muscle. For example, when your arms are down at your sides, your elbow joint is fully extended; when you bend your elbows to make your biceps bulge, your elbow joint is fully flexed. At the fully extended position, your arm cannot open any more because the bones of the upper and lower arm hit each other. At the fully flexed position, the biceps makes contact with the forearm.

No matter what speed the weight moves, each rep should be perfect. This is probably the most important lesson to take into the weight room. There should be absolutely no cheating, which follows the old saying of "quality, not quantity." Cheat reps, or shortened-range reps, decrease overall muscle involvement and decrease your muscle's ability to grow evenly. The shape of your muscle, although mostly genetic, is partially determined by the performance of each rep.

A perfect rep generally requires a two-second concentric phase followed by a three- or four-second eccentric phase of each complete rep. Once you have perfected technique, then you can increase rep speed. If you are trying to lift explosively, the weight should be light enough to do the rep properly. Before doing any advanced movements, you must master the skills of the basic exercises. In resistance training, your form should always be perfected before increasing your weight. If you use the motto that "technique comes first," you will stay injury free and see the greatest improvements.

## Grip

There are different ways to grip the bar, a handle, or your resistance tubing. In general, a thumb-lock grip, shown in figure 3.6, is the safest and most effective. You wrap your fingers around the bar and your thumb around the opposite way so that your thumb locks in against your fingers. The open grip, commonly called the false grip, has your thumb on the same side as your wrists. By not squeezing your grip tightly and resting the bar on your hands instead, you reduce the work by the forearm, but you also increase the danger considerably in that the bar or dumbbell can easily fall out of your hands. Additionally, false grips have been known to cause wrist soreness, and therefore the thumb-lock grip is best.

Along with the grip itself is the position that your hand is in during the lift. You may turn your palms out and away from you (pronated hand position) or turn your palms up and in toward you (supinated hand position) or somewhere

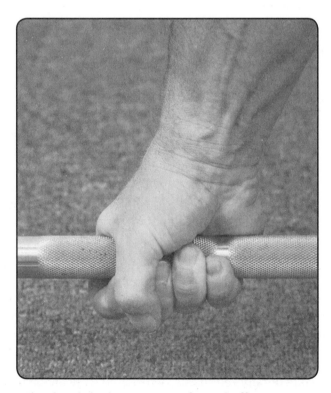

**Figure 3.6** The thumb-lock grip is a safe and effective way to grip weight equipment.

in between (neutral hand position). Hand positioning and distance, as well as foot position on lower body exercises, have considerations for both anatomy and comfort. Anatomically, changing position may change how a muscle is activated, although for the most part, the intended primary muscle of an exercise is still the most activated. From a comfort standpoint, choose the most comfortable position first, then try changing things up after you have mastered the technique.

## Spotting

Anytime you're lifting weight over your neck, a spot is a good idea. Have your partner help with lifting the bar off the rack and with re-racking when you finish your reps. The spotter should stand at the head of the bench with a solid base of support and use both legs and arms to help lift. Make sure the person spotting you is capable of lifting the entire weight if you get into real trouble. It is not recommended to have spotters at either side help with lifting unless someone is also in the middle; only very advanced lifters would require this kind of spot. Additionally, the goal of the spotter is to ensure safety and to help out if necessary. As a spotter yourself, provide enough of a spot to help but not to do all the work, unless the lifter requires more of a spot. As a lifter, if you are finding a need for a spot early on in your reps (before the last rep or two), you are lifting too heavy and should consider backing down on the weight.

# TRAINING PHILOSOPHIES

If there were only one right way to do anything, there would be no need for continued research, as we would all do the exact same thing every day. But in the true spirit of discovery, we don't believe we have found the perfect way to exercise, or for that matter, the perfect way to live healthily. In weight training, we have sound scientific principles, we have theoretical principles, and we have a few ideas for things that seem to work. And yes, there is a gray area. For the most part, we use these principles like a recipe rather than a specific set of instructions. In other words, there is room for interpretation and adjustment, like increasing spice content. And as long as you don't stray too far, you won't screw things up too badly.

## Training Movements and Muscles

Since the human body moves in many different ways and rarely by contracting only a single muscle at a time, your training program should reflect the multidimensional ways that we move and the multiple muscle actions that make it possible. The question then becomes, do we want to train movements, or do we want to train muscles? One school of thought suggests that you can mimic a particular movement by creating an exercise in the gym and training it under a loaded or resisted condition. Then when you execute the movement (e.g., while playing a sport), you will perform better. The other school of thought is to train muscles to have greater strength, power, or endurance while continuing to practice your sport movement and skills separately. Although each has merit, I support the latter approach. Train your muscles or train your sport movement and skills, but don't try to train them at the same time in the same motion. Generally, machine-based training has a fixed path of movement and focuses on muscle shape and quality, while free weights and other resistive devices have more movement options. The more movement directions or planes that a piece of equipment can provide, the more balance and control you need, which in turn requires more muscle to help stabilize the body.

Real-life movements from sports or daily activities are nearly impossible to duplicate with weight lifting. Most of our movements are reactions to previous movements, either a preconceived stimulus or one that is completely unknown. So, since we are at the mercy of something that is about to happen at every moment of every day, we need to make sure we prepare for everything, both known and unknown. That means your program should do both and use a variety of equipment to achieve a complete training program.

## Single and Multiple Sets

Without a doubt, the question of how many sets to perform has become the greatest debate in weight training. The issue is whether to follow a high-intensity training (HIT) approach, which advocates performing only one set per exercise, or a more traditional multiset approach. Without starting a full-scale war, both single-set and multiset weight training have been shown to improve strength and muscle size in all groups of people, from young adults to senior citizens and athletes alike. Although it is generally accepted that performing multiple sets produces greater gains in trained individuals, and beginners do better with single sets, several scientific research publications note that experienced lifters have shown great improvements with single-set workouts. The qualifying item probably lies within the performance of the set itself. Single and multiple sets each offer specific advantages.

In many cases, training is restricted by time. If that is the case, a one-set system may be all that can be done. Additionally, single-set exercise programs can offer more variety than a multiset program. In a multiset system you may perform the same biceps curl exercise for three or four sets, but in a single-set system you can do three or four different biceps curl exercises.

A strong argument for multiple sets is that repetitive practice is a key stimulus in making gains. Just like in sport, where you continue to practice to get better, increasing the overall amount of work you do in weight training increases your chances of making faster gains. However, if single sets are taken to failure, true overload does occur, especially if you grind out a few more reps.

If you believe the old adage that submaximal effort produces submaximal results, then any set that does not adequately tax your muscles will not produce maximal results. So if you are not working hard enough, neither is better. And once again, since your goal is the driving force behind your training program, the most logical method is a combination of both systems because some exercises may provide benefit with one set while other exercises will need multiple sets to provide any benefit.

## Max- and Single-Rep Sets

Maximum lifting implies heavy weights and only one to three repetitions per set. Maximum lifting is a good way to find your one-repetition maximum (1RM) but not a very good way to train. Furthermore, the rest time between sets needs to be long enough so that the workouts themselves have a low work output and require a long time to complete. Generally, 1RM training should be used only by trained people looking to find their true max strength or relative muscle strength or force-generating capacity. In fact, even powerlifters and Olympic lifters rarely train at pure max levels (using single reps) except in competition. A routine for strength, hypertrophy, or endurance is better suited to most people.

However, for those interested in seeing their progress, one-rep maxing does represent both a challenge and a goal that helps motivate. As long as one-rep maxes are performed infrequently and with care, they can be used as an effective training gauge. Keep in mind that in order to see continued improvement, foundational strength training using five-rep sets or greater is best. Use the following steps to find your one-repetition maximum. For safety, use a spotter or a machine. If you use a machine, your max will be 10 to 15 percent heavier than with the free weight version because the machine controls the movement, reducing the need for your body to stabilize the weight.

1. Perform one set of 10 reps with 50 percent of your estimated 1RM. Take a three-minute break.

2. Perform one set of 5 reps with 75 percent of your estimated 1RM. Take a three-minute break.

3. Perform one set of 2 reps with 85 to 90 percent of your estimated 1RM. Take a three-minute break.

4. Perform one set of 1 rep with 95 percent of your estimated 1RM. Take a three-minute break.

5. Add 5 to 10 pounds (2.5 to 5 kg) for 1 rep on each consecutive set, resting for three to five minutes between sets, until you can no longer perform the rep without help.

The major disadvantage in this type of lifting is that adaptation is mostly neurological. Lifters who perform 1RMs feel as if they are getting stronger and bigger, but the reality is that they are only weakening their overall capability. Strength and size are built by increasing total work, meaning that more reps are needed for overall improvement. Building a solid base is the most important aspect of weight training. If you perform single-rep maxes regularly, it would be like putting up roofs without a house to build them on. Furthermore, since technique is important and lifting heavy weights tends to

## NO PAIN MORE GAIN

One of the most persistent myths in strength training is that muscle soreness represents progress and that if you are not sore the next day you did not work hard enough. This is based on the notion that breaking down the muscle, causing tiny microscopic tears, is the catalyst for increasing muscle strength and size. This is an overly simplistic approach to a series of very complex physiological changes at the cellular level involving many hormones, growth factors, and nutrients. There is little scientific evidence suggesting that soreness is a true measure of training success. Although it is common to be sore for a few days when you take up a training program for the first time, attempting to be sore after every training session will quickly lead to overtraining and a variety of injuries, particularly tendinitis and joint swelling, because tendons and ligaments do not recover as quickly as muscles do from the stress of training.

encourage competition, people often lose sight of the goal of exercise in favor of throwing up big numbers. Leave the single-rep work to those competing, and if you are considering lifting as a career, get some help from an Olympic lifter or powerlifter before doing heavy-duty single-rep maxes.

## Explosive Lifting

Another hotly debated topic lies in the speed and execution of each exercise. In sport, explosive movement is a normal part of everyday life, making it obvious to some that lifting should also be explosive; however, others believe that explosive movement should be left for the playing field. This debate gives rise to two important questions. Does performing a weightlifting movement quickly build better explosive power than performing a weightlifting movement slowly? If explosive lifting does build better explosive power, does that explosive power transfer to movements out of the gym? Advocates for explosive training believe there is a direct transfer to on-field performance. Those against explosive lifting think it is dangerous and that momentum takes away from the lift itself.

In reality, both options can be beneficial, but it depends on the application and on your goal for training. If the goal of your weightlifting program is to place your muscles under tension to help them grow, then allowing other body parts to help in the lift completely degrades the value of your movement-specific repetition. In this case, explosive lifting would most likely be counterproductive. For true bodybuilding programs, slower reps would be more useful. However, this doesn't mean explosive lifting isn't valuable. In fact, I advocate explosive lifting for all people, not because there is necessarily a direct transfer to other movements, but because it teaches muscles to contract faster, which is something everyone needs given that most everyday movements take under half a second to complete (like standing up from a seated position). As you will see in chapter 15, it is wise to change up your routines every few weeks, so you may employ a few faster lifts mixed with your slower, more controlled reps.

The concerns over safety with explosive lifting are not as serious as detractors may make them seem. As with all exercises, using the proper technique is essential to ensure safety. Additionally, a proper progression from slower lifting to faster lifting should be used. Once you have control of a movement and use proper form, you can begin to move the weight quicker. When lifting fast, be careful not to lock out too quickly. At the end range of the movement, slow down and use a soft lock when fully extending the joint.

## Muscle Memory and Confusion

Your body adapts to an exercise very quickly; one of the reasons this book provides different exercises is to allow you to change them when needed. Varying the exercises will keep you from becoming bored and reduce the likelihood of overuse injuries that may occur when the same exercise is done for too long. Some people take the idea of change to the extreme and think that if the muscle gets too comfortable with a specific movement, they will not continue to see results, and thus muscle must be constantly "confused" by regularly changing up the exercises.

Since muscle does need help to remember how to do things and the catalyst for change is repetitive stimulus, changing things too frequently will actually confuse your muscles so much that they will never get good at anything—and results will take even longer. It is important to stimulate your muscles with regular exercise and allow them to get stronger and gain control of a particular movement before changing it. See the periodization section in chapter 15 to learn more about how to adjust training programs over a long period of time.

## Balance

Balance can be divided into two major subcategories: static balance and dynamic balance. Static balance, often referred to as stability, is used to hold or maintain a body position. Gymnasts use static balance to hold a cross on the rings or to support themselves on the parallel or uneven bars. A basketball or hockey player needs static balance when trying to hold a position in front of the net or in the low post. Static balance requires the ability to react to an external force that is attempting to upset your equilibrium. This requires both a high level of isometric strength as well as a certain amount of anticipation and preparation that comes with playing experience.

Dynamic balance is the ability to maintain body positions during motion and is often referred to as body control. Jumping, landing, cutting, cornering, accelerating, and decelerating all require a certain amount of balance. Athletes who have the ability to start, stop, and change direction very quickly and under control not only have excellent speed and power but also have superior dynamic balance. Dynamic balance plays an important role in injury prevention. Many knee injuries occur when the upper body continues in one direction while the lower body is going in the other direction; this causes a loss of balance and control and excessive shear or torque on the knee, resulting in an injury. Through better body control, dynamic balance helps the athlete correct body positions that may result in injury. Both static and dynamic balance should be part of a regular training program.

Balance occurs as a result of both skill training and specific balance training. Regardless of how much balance training you do, if you do not know how to move and position your body in sport or you do not possess strength from the ground up, you will never have good balance. Although balance training tends to focus on the skill itself, your training program should focus on all aspects of movement for life and sport. Spending your entire workout on an unstable surface will not meet all your needs. Furthermore, many balance training advocates believe your core is the center of movement, which is not entirely correct. It is not possible to initiate movement from the core; rather, all movement is started by the feet pressing into the ground and then continues up through a chain of linking muscle systems (called the *kinetic chain*), of which your core is the main linking system. Balance training has become synonymous with core training in popular media outlets, but really the two are independent. Often balance training has been improperly applied, causing persons to reduce the weight they use in an attempt to increase stability. The opposite should be the case—increase the weight you can handle in unstable conditions.

# 4

# WARM UP, STRETCH, COOL DOWN

Imagine going on a trip and not packing. Unless you plan to buy everything you will need while traveling, that would not be a smart choice! Before you do most tasks you prepare by getting ready. Weight training is no different. Sure you can begin lifting without warming up, but if you are well prepared, you will have a better workout. Just like giving your car a good detailing and tune-up, stretching will make your body move better and keep it healthier longer. And once you have had that perfect workout, you want those hard-earned reps to pay off, so you need to cool down to help start that recovery process sooner than later. All of these little extras help improve the overall quality and benefit of your workout and should not be left out. This chapter shows you how to keep your engine tuned and your body rolling and will help you make the most out of every workout.

## WARMING UP

The warm-up is one of the most important parts of a workout or precompetition routine. Although originally thought to primarily be a means of preventing injury, it is now commonly accepted that the main purpose of the warm-up is to improve performance, with injury prevention taking a secondary role. The positive effects of the warm-up occur because of several physiological mechanisms such as increased muscle temperature, cardiac adaptations, and injury prevention. And for athletes, the warm-up serves as mental rehearsal of the event they are about to engage in.

An increase in body temperature is one of the main physiological adaptations to warming up. Increased body temperature stimulates vasodilation (an increase in the size of arteries) in the working muscle, increasing blood flow through the muscle and improving cardiac function. In addition, the increase in body temperature speeds up nerve conduction, prepping the muscles for their upcoming task. For those with high blood pressure or other cardiac-related issues, the warm-up can prevent serious heart conditions. Instead of shocking the system with the onslaught of heavy-duty exercise, you give your heart a chance to catch up to the task slowly, decreasing the possibility of sudden heart trauma. In fact, research has shown that light jogging alone can reduce abnormal EKG readings that may arise during training since jogging slowly increases heart rate and normalizes blood flow.

Preventing injuries, such as muscle strains, may no longer be the primary purpose for warming up, but it is still a potential benefit. Most coaches agree that warming up can help prevent injuries, but most of the evidence is anecdotal, and very few, if any, studies can show that warming up decreases the incidence of musculoskeletal injuries. Since most musculoskeletal injuries occur because of strength or flexibility imbalances, and researchers cannot set up a study that would deliberately try to injure someone, it is unlikely that we will truly understand the impact of the warm-up on injury prevention. However, it seems logical that if you slowly introduce greater stress to a muscle rather than subject it to rapid punishment while cold, it will stand a better chance of both performing well and staying injury free.

For advanced athletes, the warm-up offers time to mentally prepare for battle. Many athletes talk to themselves or mimic movements they will perform during the competition. A diver may go through her rotations, and a figure skater preps for the double Axel jump. In any case, slow progressive warm-ups improve overall circulation in both athletes and beginners and prepare the body for the task while also giving athletes time to mentally focus.

For athletes and weekend warriors alike, the warm-up is crucial before exercise and sport so that you are both mentally and physically alert. The moment you are called to sprint, jump, or just move quickly, you'll be glad that you had a solid warm-up, not only to reduce the chance of injury but also to help those muscles fire more rapidly. Go to any sporting event and watch athletes before their contest. You will no doubt see most, if not all, warming up.

## Static and Dynamic Warm-Ups

When they think of warm-ups, most people figure that a light walk or jog on a treadmill should do the trick. In most cases, and especially for general activity, this would be fine. But for some people, extended warm-ups involving both stretching and specific movements may also be necessary. A static warm-up is usually in the form of stretching, although stretching alone does not really warm up the body and should really be done after the warm-up itself. Static refers to stationary, nonmoving activity, which is the norm when holding a specific stretch. Dynamic warm-ups are more common in athletic programs and include exercises such as jumping jacks, body-weight lunges or squats, and other forms of active movements. Dynamic movements are a great addition to both outdoor and home-based programs and can be used when exercising large groups or in small spaces.

## Quick Full Body Warm-Up

| | |
|---|---|
| Jumping jacks | 20 reps |
| Hamstring and lower back stretch (page 40) | 15 sec. hanging down in a forward bend |
| Lunge and reach (page 44) | 5 reps per leg |
| Quadriceps stretch (page 39) | 15 sec. per leg |
| Stationary inchworm (page 47) | 10 reps (out and back makes 1 rep) |
| Pec stretch (page 41) | 15 sec. (against wall) |
| Lateral push-up walk (page 48) | 5 reps (5 hand steps out and back makes 1 rep) |
| Upper back stretch (page 43) | 15 sec. (with partner or grabbing on to pole) |
| Overhead squat (page 47) | 10 reps (with any stick or body bar) |

## Exercise Sets as a Warm-Up

A warm-up for strength training should not only include some form of mild exercise to elevate heart rate but also prepare the muscles for the weight they are about to lift. You can warm up with resistance tubing or body weight. If you are lifting heavier weight, it is best to do some light calisthenic exercises, such as push-ups or body-weight squats, or some light resistance rows before you begin your heavy sets. If you are doing a true heavyweight strength workout, then performing a set or two of the movement with lighter weight is also recommended. For example, if you are going to do the bench press exercise, a warm-up set with 50 percent of the weight you plan to use for your workout sets is advised. Don't shock the muscle with a heavy weight; a quick warm-up set will prep your neurological system and let the muscles know what they are about to get into.

## STRETCHING

During a stretch, the muscle is elongated past its normal resting length. This loosens up the muscle, which has become tight during rest. Before any type of exercise, a good stretch will help the muscles get ready by keeping them from cramping or tightening. Stretching is also a good indicator of residual soreness or injury. If stretching causes sharp pain, or if you cannot stretch as far as usual, then avoid exercising that muscle group. Be sure to stretch only after performing a good warm-up or cool-down. Never stretch a cold muscle.

Always stretch all muscles before and after exercise, whether or not that muscle group is being trained. Often a muscle will tighten up or spasm in a part of the body other than the area being trained, causing discomfort. For example, the hamstrings may cramp up while the lifter performs a bench press. Cramping in an area not being worked often occurs during weightlifting because, as the body strains to lift the weight, muscles other than those directly involved in the lift tighten up to help the body create the necessary force.

## ARE YOU DOUBLE JOINTED?

The term *double jointed* means that someone has a large range of motion at a joint. No one really has two joints in one place. Generally, a double-jointed person is able to hyperextend a joint without someone else's help, causing an exaggerated stretch of the muscle and joint.

The main muscle groups that need to be considered in a stretching routine are the quadriceps, hamstrings, groin (adductors and abductors), lower back, triceps, and pectoralis major and minor (pecs). Secondary areas include the calves (especially if you jog), neck, shins, biceps, forearms, latissimus dorsi (upper back), and the joints of the ankle, wrists, knees, and shoulders. Ideally, you should stretch all muscles every day. However, if time is limited, stretching only the primary muscles is fine. Be sure to stretch muscles you are training both before and after your workout.

A good warm-up stretching routine does not need to take long, but it must incorporate all the major muscle groups in the body. Whether you use static or dynamic stretching, the routine should take only 10 minutes at the most. Before stretching an injured area, consult your physician; stretching and exercising an injured area may not be wise.

In the past few years, stretching has gained much attention in the athletic community. Many kinds of stretches can be performed, but they all fall under three main categories: static, dynamic, and ballistic. In static stretching, you move to a joint's maximum range and hold the stretch for as little as 2 seconds to as long as 60 seconds. A dynamic stretch slowly moves through a stretched position and can be done passively (without help) or actively (with help). The move from an unstretched position to the maximum stretched position usually takes about 10 to 20 seconds. Ballistic stretching uses a bouncing motion to move from an unstretched position to a stretched position. This method of stretching is used by athletes and advanced lifters; beginners should avoid it until they have developed sound stretching technique. At first, ballistic stretching should be attempted only with supervision. Once technique is mastered, progress from your dynamic stretch to a more explosive stretch a little at a time rather than just going full bore and risking injury.

New research suggests that ballistic stretching may be more beneficial than static stretching before a strength training session, and some researchers have speculated that static stretches may actually weaken your strength. However, much research still reports the benefits of static stretching. Since the science is not conclusive at this point, your best option is to use a dynamic warm-up that includes static stretching. This way you get the best of both worlds: improvements in flexibility over time from static stretching and preparation of the neurological system for fast muscle firing from ballistic stretching.

# STATIC STRETCHES

For static stretches, you slowly move into the stretch position (the point where you feel slight tenderness or pain) for a given muscle and hold it for 10 to 30 seconds. Some stretching advocates recommend holding a stretch for 60 seconds or more, but there is no proof that longer is better. Overtime, you will become more flexible, and you will be able to increase your range of motion. During a stretch itself, you may feel your muscles loosen up, and you may be able to stretch a little further.

## Calf Stretch

Lean forward against a wall with your legs in lunge position. Bend your front leg and place your weight on it. Stretch the back of your back leg, keeping your back heel on the ground. This stretch also stretches the hip flexors.

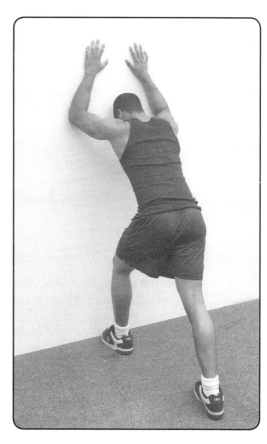

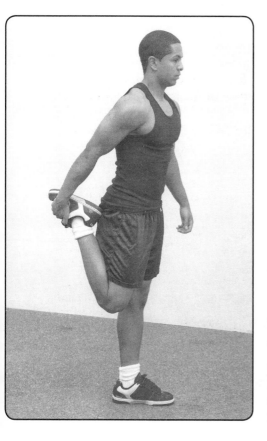

## Quadriceps Stretch

You can do this stretch either standing or lying on your belly. Bend your knee and grab your foot, pulling your heel to your buttocks. For an advanced stretch for your rectus femoris and hip flexors, pull your leg back during the stretch.

## Hamstring and Lower Back Stretch

Sit on the ground with one leg extended and the other bent, the bottom of your foot touching the knee of your extended leg. This is the modified hurdler position. Reach toward the foot of your extended leg, tucking your head down. For an additional calf stretch, grab hold of the toes of your extended leg, and pull back on them as you stretch forward.

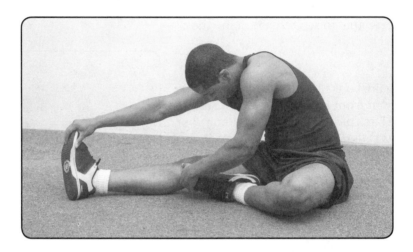

## Groin Stretch

Sit on the ground with the bottoms of your feet touching each other. Press your knees down with your elbows as you pull your heels toward your groin.

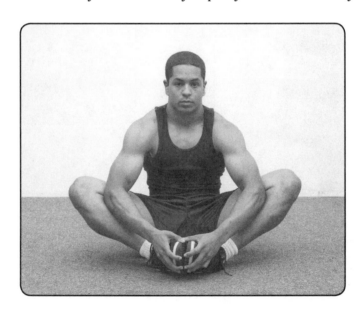

## Hip Flexor Stretch

This is an advanced stretch. Kneel with one knee on the ground and the other knee bent, with the foot flat. Lean toward the front leg. Keep the upper body upright or even slightly backward. For added stretch, press your hands against the knee, pushing your upper body backward.

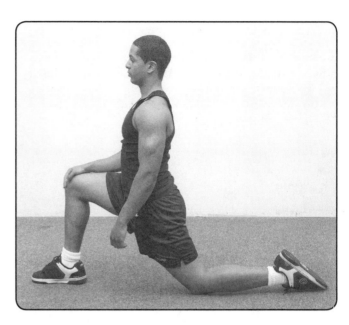

## Pec Stretch

Stand next to a wall, in a doorway, or next to a machine. Extend your arm to the side and contact the wall, doorframe, or machine with your hand. Lean forward to get a stretch through the pectoralis major by creating resistance against your hand.

## Triceps Stretch

Raise your arm overhead, flex your elbow, and reach down your back. Use your other arm to pull back on the elbow for additional stretch.

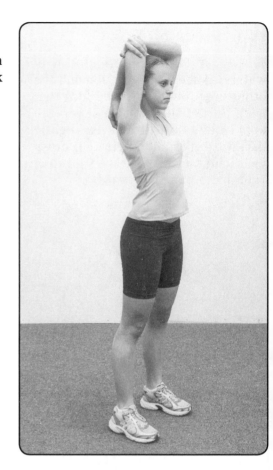

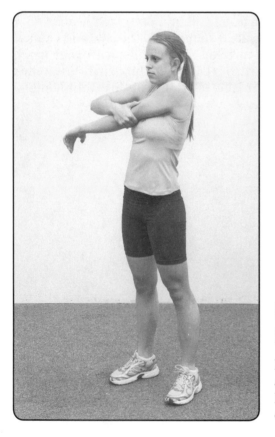

## Rear Deltoid and Upper Back Stretch

Reach across your body at chest height with one arm. Grab that arm at the elbow with your other hand, and continue to pull your arm across your chest.

## Upper Back Stretch

Stand upright about 3 feet (1 m) in front of a pole or machine. Reach out and grab the pole or machine with both hands, bending at the waist. Press down on the pole or machine, stretching your upper back. This will also stretch your pecs.

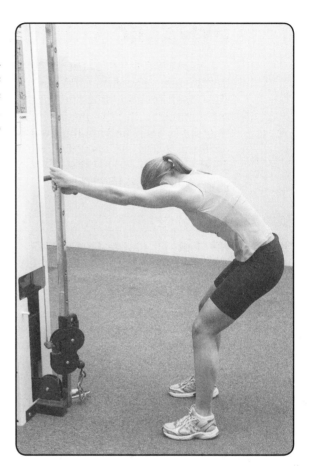

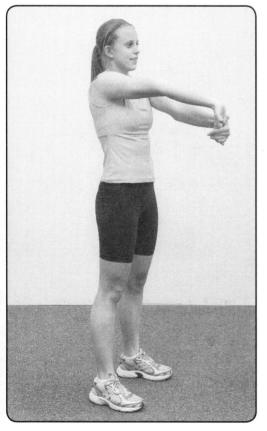

## Biceps Stretch

Fully extend your arm out in front, with your palm and forearm turned up. With your other hand, grab the hand of the outstretched arm, and gently pull back on your fingers.

# DYNAMIC STRETCHES

A dynamic stretch uses the same basic principles as the static stretch except that instead of holding the stretch, you move back and forth between the start position and your end range in a slow controlled fashion. The general recommendation is to perform 5 to 10 reps per stretch. Some exercises in this book, such as walking lunges, are similar to dynamic stretches when performed with no weight. Long range of motion dynamic stretches make good warm up moves if you are going to do faster paced, less controlled activity like playing a sport.

## Lunge and Reach

Start with your legs split forward to back about three feet (1 m) apart. Begin by descending until your lead leg is parallel with the ground. As you descend to your lunge position, raise your arms over your head as far as possible. Stand back up, bringing your arms back down. This can be done while walking or stationary, and a rotation component can be added by twisting the upper body at the waist.

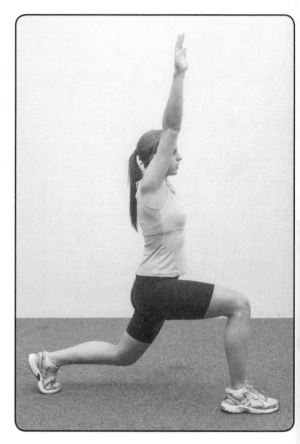

## Knee-to-Chest Walk

Stand facing the direction you intend to walk. Shift your weight to your left leg. Pull up on your right knee, bringing it to your chest. Hold the position for a second before returning to the start. Take a step forward, and repeat on the opposite leg. Keep your head and chest up, looking forward and maintaining an erect posture. For an extra challenge, you can extend up onto the toe of your standing leg while holding the other leg at your chest.

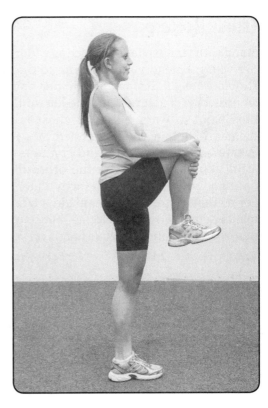

## Chain Breakers

Stand with your feet slightly wider than shoulder-width apart. Extend your arms out as far as possible to your sides at shoulder height. In a deliberate moderate-speed motion, squeeze your arms together, coming across your chest until they cross completely so that your left arm is past your right shoulder and vice versa. Squeeze at the fully closed position, then open back up to the start.

## Trunk Rotations

Stand with your feet about twice as wide as shoulder width. Extend your arms out to the sides at shoulder height. Rotate your upper body as far as possible (90 degrees) to the left so that your hips point forward but your chest is perpendicular. Maintain your extended arm position. Rotate back to the start, and continue past for a full 180-degree twist in the other direction. Continue rotating back and forth under control. For a greater stretch you can add a trunk bend, making complete body circles, but you may be more comfortable with your hands on your hips.

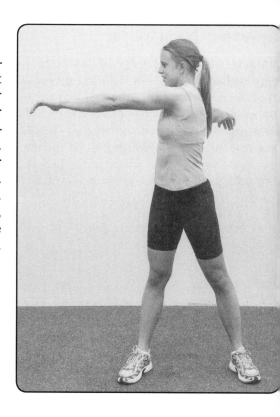

## Duck Walk

Start by standing tall with your feet about shoulder-width apart and your hands locked behind your head. Squat down as far as possible (keeping your hands behind your head). From this deep squat position, stay low and walk forward. For an added challenge, you can rotate 90 degrees in either direction and walk sideways.

# Overhead Squat

Start by standing tall with your feet about shoulder-width apart and arms fully extended overhead. Squat down as deep as possible, pressing your arms upward to maximize your stretch. Stand back up and repeat. Maintain a tight torso position throughout the movement.

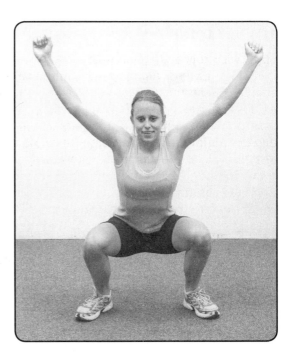

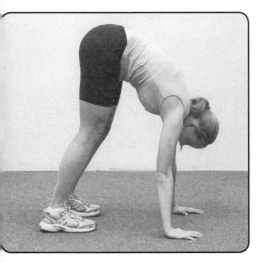

# Stationary Inchworm

Start in the push-up position. Keeping your legs fixed and straight the entire time, "walk" your hands backward toward your feet, sticking your butt into the air. Get as close as you can to your feet with your legs straight, then walk your hands back out to the starting position. Repeat for 10 reps. For an added challenge, continue moving by walking forward as you come back up.

## Lateral Push-Up Walk

Start in a regular push-up position. Keep your feet fixed to the floor in the same position. Shuffle your hands five "steps" to the left while pivoting on your fixed feet. "Walk" back to the center, then take five "steps" to the right and then back to the center. Repeat for 10 reps on each side. You can also perform this exercise while allowing your feet to move. Shuffle with both your arms and feet five full steps in each direction. Keep your torso tight during the entire exercise.

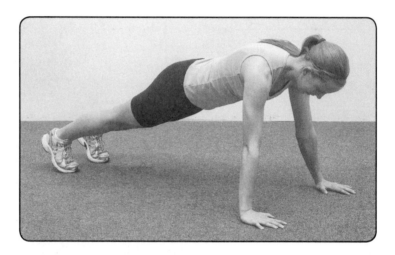

## Mountain Climbers

Start in the push-up position. Keep your torso tight and arms fully extended. Keeping your left leg extended, bring your right knee up to your side even with your chest while staying parallel with the ground. Move your right leg back to the start position while simultaneously bringing your left knee up to your chest. Keep an even, slow pace.

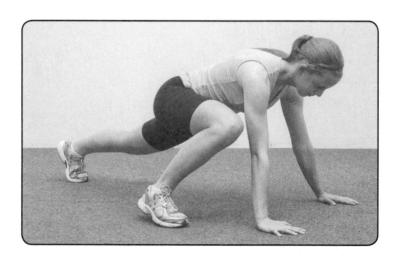

# Spider-Man

Using the mountain climber position, step forward with one leg but instead of bringing your knee even with your chest, bring it outside your shoulder. As your knee reaches your armpit, walk your opposite hand forward while pressing back on the front leg. At the same time, move your opposite leg up toward its same-side armpit while extending the other leg backward. This is a difficult warm-up exercise to get the hang of, as it demands core strength to keep your body parallel to the ground.

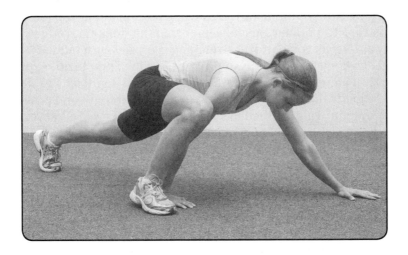

## WEIGHT TRAINING AND FLEXIBILITY

Flexibility is usually defined as the range of motion about a joint or group of joints in a system. This definition is somewhat inadequate, however. Joint range is based on bone shape and the stretch and pliability of connective tissues (cartilage, tendons, and ligaments). Although part of your ability to be flexible is genetic, you can become more flexible through a dedicated, regular routine of stretches. Stretching slowly increases the range of motion about the joint.

Contrary to popular belief, weight training does not reduce flexibility as long as you perform stretching exercises on a regular basis. Weight training may actually improve flexibility if practiced regularly because it increases the strength and pliability of tendons, ligaments, and the joints themselves. It increases muscle strength and prevents injury by improving the tendon's ability to stretch as well as increasing its strength, which prevents tearing and overrotation or dislocation of a joint. Weight training also helps increase the tendon's ability to return to its normal shape after deformation. Think of a rubber band that, over time, loses its ability to return to its original shape after being stretched. Training keeps tendons pliable over time so they return to their resting length after being stretched.

Resistance training will help you bring the area of the body being stretched into position and hold the position. Without muscle strength and endurance, you can't hold the position as long. Weight training decreases the chances of injury during flexibility training, but remember, no form of training can prevent all injuries.

# COOLING DOWN

If you finish your workout and your heart rate is still elevated, it is a good idea to bring it back down slowly. A cool-down increases the body's ability to return to normal after exercise by preventing the blood from pooling in certain areas. If you have ever gotten dizzy when standing up (known as orthostatic hypotension), it is because your blood has pooled in your lower body, leaving the brain in demand for some oxygen. Although this is normally nothing to worry about, it can be dangerous, as some people have passed out while trying to stand up. A safe way to bring your exercise heart rate back down is to do a cool-down.

Your cool-down can be similar to your warm-up. Perform 5 to 10 minutes of a slow, rhythmic exercise, followed by 10 minutes of a full-body stretching routine. For example, a light bike ride and stretch make a perfect end to a hard workout.

# 5

# CHEST

One of the most noticeable parts of the body, the chest is responsible for many arm movements such as throwing, pushing, and hitting. A strong, well-defined chest is the hallmark of a great training program. The major chest muscles are the pectoralis major and pectoralis minor. These strong muscles move the arms across the body and toward the waist. The pecs allow for several different movements, and there are several different ways to strengthen them.

All pressing movements require your pecs, triceps, and anterior deltoids to play a role in the movement. So trying to isolate your pecs is not always easy. That also means that grouping exercises together to prevent overtraining will be an important part of your workout week. If you really want great upper body development, you will need to use both the pressing movements and the isolated pec exercises found in this chapter.

The main lift, and perhaps the single most practiced exercise, is the bench press. No other exercise is more heralded than this spectacle of strength and prowess. The bench press works not only the pecs but also several other muscles. In addition to developing the chest, the bench press helps develop many of the muscles that act on the shoulder joint, including the anterior deltoid and the triceps.

# Bench Press

The motion of the bench press resembles an upside-down push-up. This exercise requires a great deal of concentration and arm coordination. Though the free weight version of the bench press is described here, some gyms may have a machine bench press option. It is important that you follow proper technique and start with a weight you can handle.

1. Lie on the weight bench. Grab the bar, hands shoulder-width or a little wider apart. Keep your feet on the floor. Keep your shoulders, buttocks, and head against the bench at all times. To relieve the pressure on your lower back, it should have a slight arch. You should be able to slide your hand under your lower back.

2. Inhale deeply, and remove the bar from the rack. Pause for two counts, then begin to lower the weight toward your chest.

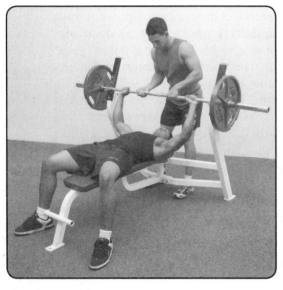

Starting position

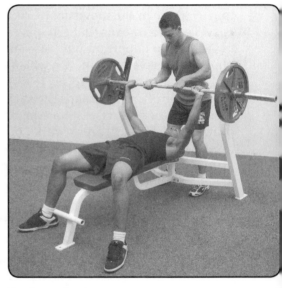

Remove the bar

3. Lower the bar steadily, and pause for two counts when it touches your chest. The bar should cross at or slightly above your nipples.

4. To begin the ascent, rapidly drive the weight up, maintaining a constant speed. Exhale as you lift the weight. Continue to lift the weight until your arms are fully extended. The bar will naturally follow an arc and end up just over your neck. Although many people think locking the arms is bad, it is important to move the bar through the complete range of motion. A gentle lock is acceptable and ensures that you have completed the upward motion.

There are several variations of the bench press and many other chest exercises. Each exercise works the pecs and supporting muscles slightly differently. Remember, specificity requires that you choose exercises that reflect your needs and goals.

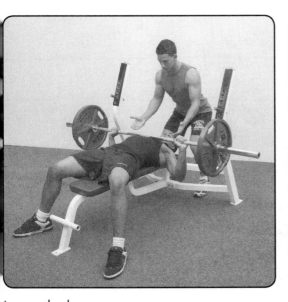

Lower the bar

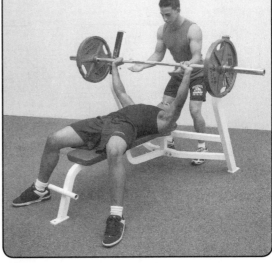

Extend your arms

## Incline Bench Press

The incline press works the upper pecs a little more than the flat bench press.

1. Set the bench at about a 45-degree angle. Decreasing the angle puts more emphasis on the middle chest and front shoulders; increasing the angle puts more emphasis on the upper chest and middle shoulders and triceps.

2. Lower and raise the weight as you did in the bench press. The bar should touch a little higher on your chest, near your collarbone.

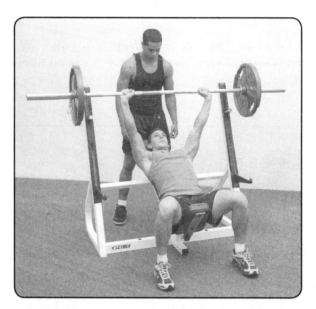

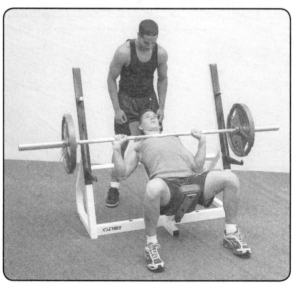

# Dumbbell Bench Press

This movement emphasizes the muscles that help stabilize the shoulders. The weights will feel awkward when you do the dumbbell bench press for the first time. Controlling them is the key.

1. Lie on your back on a flat bench. Dig your shoulders into the bench, and pull your shoulder blades together. This tightens your body, lending additional support to the shoulders.
2. Start with a dumbbell in each hand, palms turned forward, the dumbbells over your chest, and your elbows away from your body.
3. Press the dumbbells by extending your arms.
4. Lower the dumbbells back to the starting position. If you feel the dumbbells getting squirrelly on you, try to bring the dumbbells together when you press them.

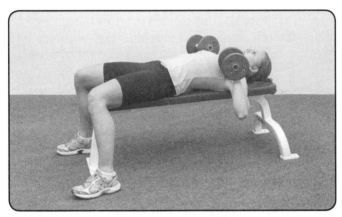

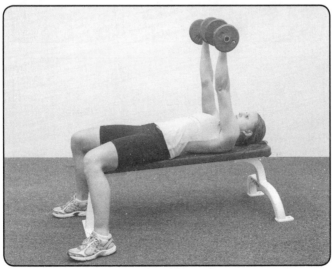

## Single-Arm Bench Press

When looking to increase your challenge, try performing single-arm variations of the flat and incline bench presses. When using dumbbells, the bench press starts at the chest, unlike the barbell version, which comes off the rack.

1. To get the dumbbells to the starting position, rest the dumbbells on your knees while you are seated at the end of the bench. Lie backward on the bench, and pull the dumbbells while simultaneously raising your knees up to push the dumbbells back toward you as you lie down. Tighten your torso, and use the same body position as for the incline press.

2. While keeping one dumbbell on your chest, press the other one straight up until your arm is fully extended. Pause for two counts then lower.

3. You have the option of alternating arms or completing all your reps with one arm first. Generally, alternating ensures that both arms fatigue at a similar rate.

For a more difficult challenge, instead of resting the nonmoving dumbbell at your chest, try keeping it locked out at arm's length while pressing and lowering the other dumbbell. To alternate this version, start by pressing both dumbbells up, then lowering and raising one, then lowering and raising the other.

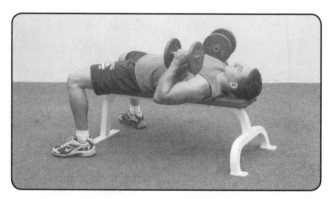

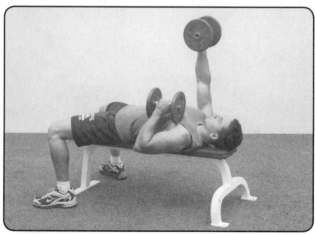

# Unstable Bench Press

Unstable training is more sport specific and for advanced lifters, but trying these same lifts on a stability ball will increase your challenge significantly. Although some people use this exercise for core development, the added difficulty is at your shoulder girdle and will both train and challenge your rotator cuff muscles. Remember, though, if your goal is to increase pec size and strength, training on an unstable surface is not the way to go. Also, before you attempt to do any move on an unstable surface, you should be able to perform its stable version flawlessly.

1. Start by grabbing a pair of dumbbells (use lighter ones than you would use on a stable surface) and sitting at the base of a stability ball.

2. Bring the dumbbells up to shoulder height. Walk your feet out from the stability ball so that you make a bridge, with your shoulders and back on the ball, your torso extended, and your feet flat on the ground, your knees at 90 degrees.

3. Press the dumbbells up to arm's length while maintaining a tight torso. Hold for two counts and bring back down. You can perform single-arm versions of this exercise as well.

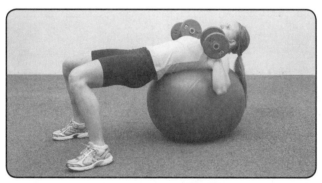

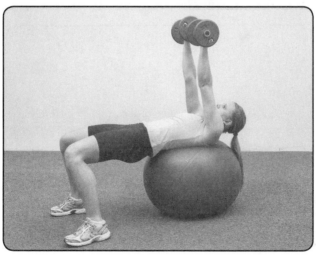

## Cable (or Machine) Pec Fly

The pec fly is another exercise that isolates the pecs. It allows for greater range of motion than the bench press. With the cable or machine fly, the arms are extended out to the sides at chest height, with the elbows straight out or bent 90 degrees depending on the machine you are using.

1. If you are using a cable machine or your machine has handles, grab the handles and extend your arms leaving a slight bend at the elbow. For a machine with pads, turn your palms so they face forward, and place your arms against the pads so that your lower arm, hands, and elbows are in complete contact..

2. Squeeze the handles or pads toward each other, applying equal force to both. In the fully contracted position, the handles or pads should come directly in front of you. (Touching them together is fine.)

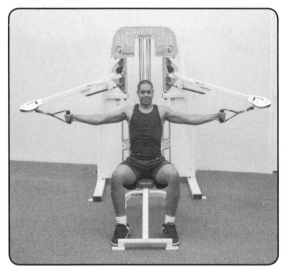 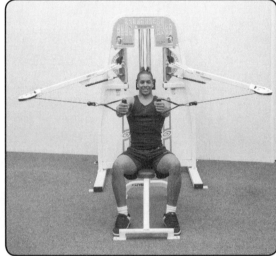

# Dumbbell Pec Fly

The dumbbell pec fly is more difficult than the machine pec fly because it requires you to stabilize your upper body and create the path the dumbbells follow rather than having a fixed line.

1. Lie on a flat weight bench with your arms fully extended over your chest. With the dumbbells in your hands, turn your palms inward and touch the dumbbells together.
2. Keeping a slight bend in your elbows, pull the dumbbells apart until your upper arms are parallel to the ground.
3. Pause for two counts at the bottom position.
4. Using a bear-hugging motion, return the dumbbells to the top.

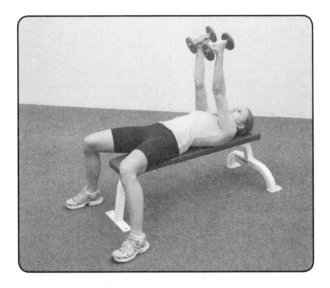

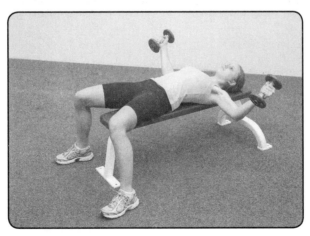

# Cable Cross

The cable cross is perhaps the most flamboyant of chest exercises. It is a good way to work the pecs and can be performed one arm at a time.

1. Stand in the middle of the cable machine, with arms extended to the sides at shoulder height. Position one foot ahead of the other to create stability.
2. Grab the machine handles, palms down, and pull toward the middle of your body, keeping your elbows slightly bent. Keep a slight bend in your knees, and lean slightly forward.
3. Cross palms or bring your hands together about 6 to 12 inches (15 to 30 cm) in front of your belly button.
4. Release the handles upward and backward to return to the starting position.

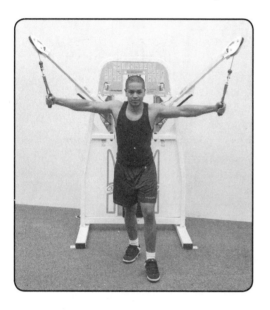 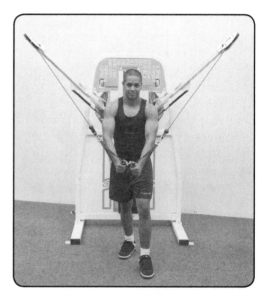

## — TAKE IT TO THE GYM

### Train Smart

Veteran bench pressers know a few tricks for successful benching. The ultimate goal, especially for men, is to load up the plates, trying to hit the legendary three-plate pinnacle—three 45-pound (20 kg) plates per side, plus the 45-pound bar, totaling 315 pounds (140 kg). Although that may not be in your sights now, it may be in your future. Don't try to lift like the veterans until your technique is solid and you have developed sufficient strength.

Grip all barbells and dumbbells in a monkey grip, with your thumb wrapped around the bar or dumbbell. Placement of your hands on the bar is also important. Generally, a narrow grip involves the triceps more, whereas a wider grip involves more of the pecs.

The key to good technique is to get into a solid, tight position on the bench. Keep your body in contact with the bench throughout the entire pressing movement. Use your feet for support; placing them on the bench reduces stability and decreases the emphasis on the working muscles. Position your feet a little wider than shoulder-width apart and slightly back. Pull your shoulders back to form a solid base, and keep them in check throughout the movement.

Control the descent of the weight. A controlled descent allows the muscles to build up elastic energy that will help lift the bar back up. As you begin to drive the weight up, push your body back into the bench and flatten your shoulders. Don't bounce the weight off your chest or use momentum to move the weight, as this can lead to injury and loss of control.

## — TRAIN AT HOME

### Practice Your Push-Ups

If you are not heading down to the gym and still want to get a great workout for your chest, you have several ways to do it in your own home. First, never forget the power of your own body weight as resistance. Push-ups are great standbys and still used in most strength programs. If you are very strong, try elevating your legs by putting them on a bench or chair so that more body weight is forward. Another great way to increase the difficulty is to perform the reps with your hands very close together or very wide apart.

If you have difficulty with regular push-ups, you can modify the push-up to make it easier. To reduce the amount of body weight you must support, place your feet on the floor and your hands on a chair or on a step to take a more upright position. If you want to increase the challenge, you can use a balance disc or med ball as the base support for your hands. This method allows you to target the same muscles and perform the same general movement. This is a great addition at the gym as well. And if you have resistance tubing, fix the middle of the tubing around a bedpost or banister, grab the handles with your back against the rail, and perform your reps standing up. Special resistance tubing is available that can be hooked to a doorknob.

# CREATE A CHEST ROUTINE

The bench press is a great stand-alone exercise, but when it's combined with other exercises, you can reach new levels in chest development. The bench press is easily coupled with the pec fly. To show your pecs who's boss, try a pre- or postexhaust training routine (see page 188 and 189). Simply perform a set of pec flys immediately before (preexhaust) or after (postexhaust) the bench press. Allow only enough rest between exercises to move to the next exercise.

For additional variety, try alternating between exercises within your workout or within your training week. For example, perform flat bench presses one workout and incline bench presses the next. Perform cable crosses between bench presses and incline presses. The combinations are limited only by your imagination. The bench press incorporates so many muscles that you are bound to work your chest well. Remember, muscles will begin to tire when you perform multiple sets of several exercises. Adjust your weights accordingly.

Don't be afraid to change things. You don't always have to start with the bench press on Monday. Try one of the popular combinations shown in the table. Routine 1 is good for general fitness, routine 2 is appropriate for strength development, and routine 3 is a good change of pace.

| Exercise | Number of sets | Reps per set | Rest between sets |
|---|---|---|---|
| **Routine 1** | | | |
| Bench press | 2 | 12 | 90 sec. |
| Incline bench press | 2 | 10 | 90 sec. |
| Cable cross | 2 | 12 | 60 sec. |
| **Routine 2** | | | |
| Dumbbell pec fly | 2 | 12 | 90 sec. |
| Bench press | 2 | 10 | 90 sec. |
| Single-arm bench press | 2 | 10 | 90 sec. |
| **Routine 3** | | | |
| Incline bench press | 2 | 10 | 90 sec. |
| Dumbbell pec fly | 2 | 12 | 60 sec. |
| Dumbbell bench press | 3 | 15 | 90 sec. |

# 6

# BACK

One important strategy for weight training is to balance your muscle building to prevent orthopedic problems. Therefore, while training the chest, it is essential to train the back as well. Upper back exercises involve pulling movements. In all pulling movements, the latissimus dorsi (lats), rhomboids, trapezius (traps), rear deltoids, and teres major are worked, as well as the biceps and other arm flexors. In fact, many routines incorporate both upper back and biceps work on the same day. When working the back, concentrate on initiating all movements with the back muscles and not the biceps. Biceps involvement is inevitable, however, and so you should account for this when you plan your exercises so you do not overwork your biceps. Consider working your biceps on the same day as your back, or allow for plenty of recovery between your back day and your biceps training day.

Since pulling movements are a function of many muscles and not just the lats, the decision of where to place your hands and how the movement should be performed will control how your back is isolated and whether or not your biceps or rear deltoids contribute. The more help the movement gets from other muscles, the less likely you are to isolate the lats. This is both good and bad. If you are looking to improve lat size and shape, then you should choose more isolation exercises; if you are looking more for sport performance improvement, you should welcome the additional arm activity to help increase pulling strength.

The main exercise for the upper back is the seated row, which is the perfect complement to the bench press. Proper execution of this lift will not only help with anchoring a tug-of-war contest but also improve your overall upper body shape.

## Seated Row

For maximal lat involvement, the seated row is best performed using a cable system. However, upright machines offer stability and some offer lower back support, making them slightly easier to train with for beginners. Your initial hand position will dictate which muscles you emphasize. With your arms beside you and your elbows in close, you will emphasize the lat muscles slightly more. If you use a bar attachment on the cable, placing your elbows out to the sides (armpits forming a 90-degree angle), you will place greater emphasis on the rear deltoids and rhomboids. In either case, all muscles are worked in every position, and the actual movement itself remains the same.

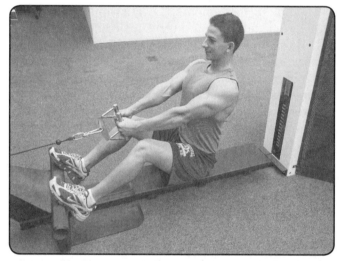

Cable machine starting position

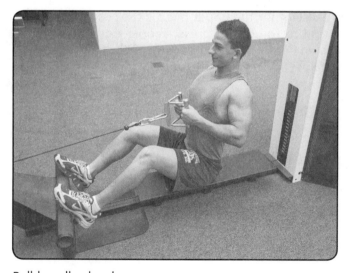

Pull handles back

1. Concentrate on your body position. Get yourself properly set in the machine. Make sure your form is tight. Plant your feet firmly on the ground or against the supports to increase your stability (your balance or ability to control the weight). Since the cable machine provides no support for your upper body, you must keep your body positioned correctly. Look forward, and sit upright with your chest out. Contract your abs, and do not bend at the waist. The handles should be at arm's length when your arms are completely extended.

2. Grab the handles and slowly pull them to your chest. During the movement, pull your shoulder blades together.

3. Pull back as far as you can, then pause for two counts. Do not use the momentum created by bending at your waist to pull the handles back.

4. Return the weight to the starting position by slowly allowing the weight to extend your arms. Fight against the resistance as your arms extend.

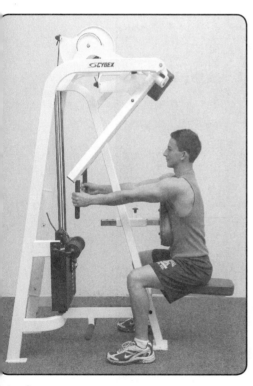

Machine starting position

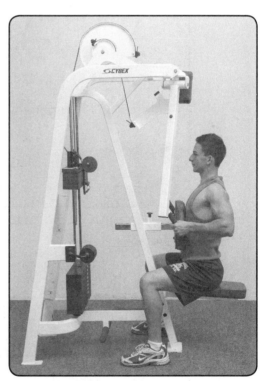

Pull handles back

## Dumbbell Row

A great way to isolate your lats, focus on form, and create better overall upper back development is to use a dumbbell and concentrate on one arm at a time.

1. Rest your right hand and knee on a flat bench, in line about two feet (.6 m) apart. Use your left leg to keep your balance. Keep a straight back, eyes looking at the ground. Do not raise your head.
2. Grab the dumbbell with your left hand, arm extended.
3. Pull up and back, keeping your upper arm tight to your left side as you pull the weight up to your waist. The motion is similar to sawing wood.
4. Slowly extend your left arm, returning the dumbbell to the starting position. Do not jerk the weight up or rotate the body during the lift. If this happens, you are lifting too much weight.

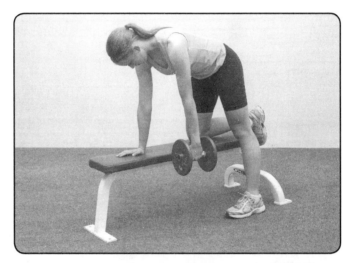

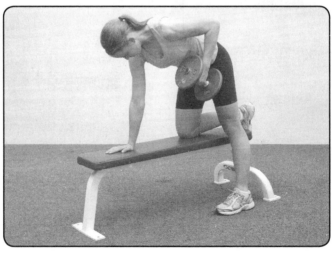

## Lat Pull-Down

The primary variation of the seated row is the lat pull-down, which—you guessed it—works the lats.

1. Sit in a lat pull-down machine with your arms extended overhead. Hold the bar in a monkey grip, hands about twice shoulder-width apart, palms turned away from you. Your arms should form a V overhead. Lean slightly back from the waist to prevent hitting yourself in the head with the bar.
2. Bring the bar down to the top of your chest. (Some lifters pull the bar behind their heads, but this position often compromises the upper neck and causes the lower back to round. Both are major flaws. If you choose to pull the bar behind your head, maintain proper position by keeping your chest up and your head facing forward.)
3. Return the bar to the starting position.

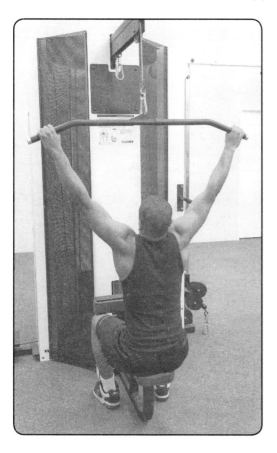
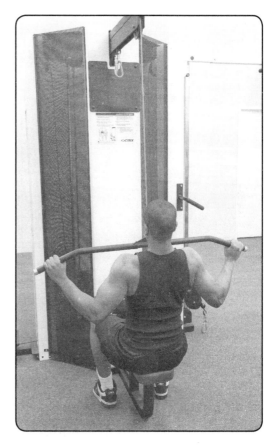

## Chin-Up

Another variation is the chin-up.

1. Hang from a chin-up bar, arms fully extended, palms turned toward you. Your elbows should be in direct line with your shoulders. Your hands should grip the bar about shoulder-width apart.

2. Pull yourself up so that your chin passes the bar and your collarbone (or clavicle) is nearly even with the bar.

3. Slowly lower your body to the starting point. If you have trouble lifting your body weight, then perform front pulls. Work on full range of motion, and in time, you will be able to chin your body.

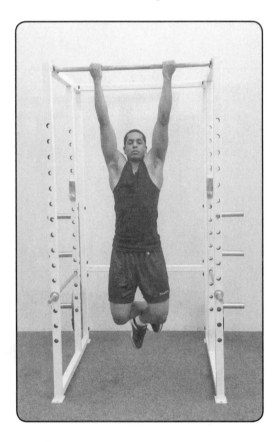 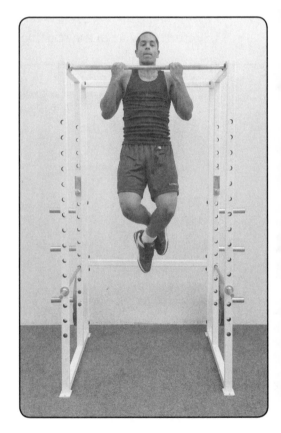

# Front Pull

If you have trouble chinning your body, try the front pull on a lat pull-down machine.

1. Sit in the machine. Grab the overhead bar, arms fully extended, palms turned toward you, hands about shoulder-width apart.

2. Pull the bar past your chin and down toward your collarbone, hold for a brief moment (or a two count), then slowly return the bar to the start by fully extending your arms.

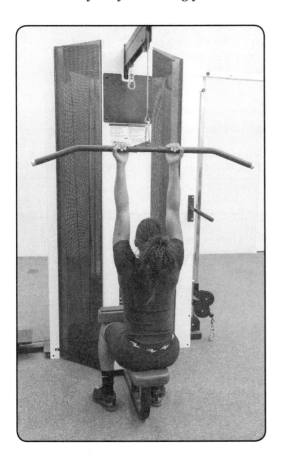
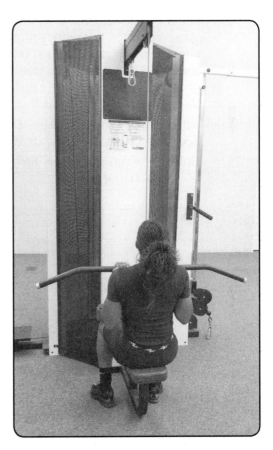

## Dumbbell Pullover

Another great exercise is the pullover. The dumbbell pullover requires paying strict attention to form. This is an isolation movement; the only joint that should move is the shoulder. Throughout the exercise, keep your arms extended, with elbows slightly bent. Do not flex and extend your elbows during the movement.

1. Stand a dumbbell on the floor at the head of a weight bench. Lie on the bench with your head at the end near the dumbbell. Reach back and grab the dumbbell with both hands, elbows slightly bent. The dumbbell should be about even with your head at the starting position with your arms extended but with a slight bend in the elbows. (The initial movement to raise the dumbbell from the floor to the starting position may be a bit difficult. You can pull your arms in to get the dumbbell off the ground.)

2. Pull the dumbbell over your face. For obvious reasons, it is wise to have a firm grip on the dumbbell. The dumbbell will track in an arc from the floor to a position over your face.

3. Hold for two counts at the top before returning slowly and under control to your starting position.

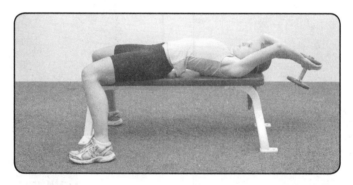

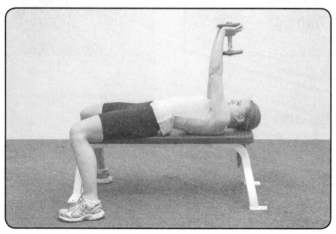

# Straight-Arm Pull-Down

If you want to isolate your lats, virtually eliminating biceps muscles, this exercise is your answer.

1. Stand straight up (with a slight bend in your knees) facing a high pulley system with a straight bar attachment. Fully extend your arms overhead (taking a step or two backward if needed), and grab the bar with an open grip, palms facing down.

2. Pull the bar to shoulder height, with your arms fully extended in front of you. Keeping your arms locked (elbows completely extended), pull down toward your body. Start with light weight, and get used to the movement and body position. Don't shrug or push with your arms; instead, try to isolate the lats and pull the bar down toward your waist.

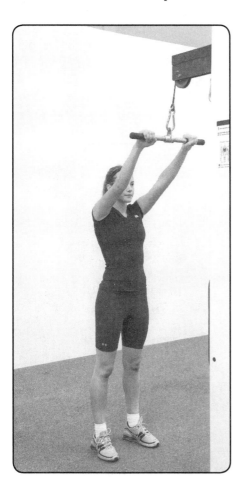 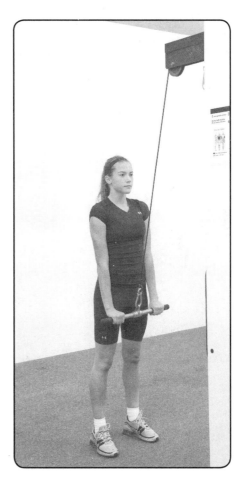

## Bent-Over Barbell Row

If you want to take your training to a new level, try this pure strength move commonly used by athletes and bodybuilders. You will need an Olympic barbell to get the most out of this exercise.

1. Start by standing with your feet slightly wider than shoulder width, with the barbell across your shins. Reach down and grab the barbell with a thumb-lock grip, palms facing backward. (For an even greater challenge, try the reverse-grip version, where you use a palms forward hand position to emphasize the biceps' contribution to the pulling motion.)

2. Stand up with the weight, give a slight bend in the knees, and lean forward so that your torso is just above parallel with the ground.

3. Pull the bar to your waist by squeezing your shoulder blades together (retracting the scapulae, or contracting your rhomboids) and contracting your lats. As you pull upward, your elbows should flare out to the sides between 45 and 60 degrees. Your full rep is complete when the barbell touches your upper abdomen.

4. Lower the bar under control while exhaling.

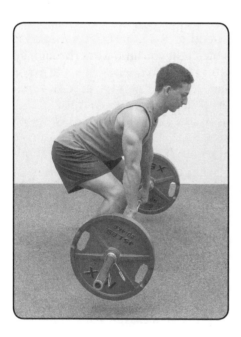 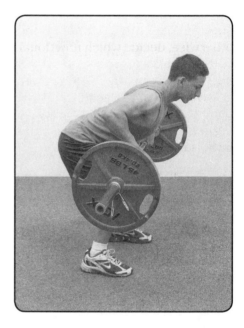

# TAKE IT TO THE GYM

## Earn Your Wings

Lifters who have exceptionally large, flared out, V-shaped lats are said to have "bat wings," referring to the way a bat's wings flare to the side. To truly develop bat wings, focus on your back. A trick used by many lifters is to retract the scapulae (pull the shoulder blades together) before initiating the movement. By doing this, you not only involve the tough-to-work rhomboids but also position the lats so they bear the load more evenly and decrease biceps involvement. Concentrate on initiating the movement with your upper back.

Deciding whether to keep your arms in or out and which grip to use is more a decision of outcome and function than comfort. If you want to develop lats more fully, you need to increase the range of motion as much as possible and reduce the reliance on your biceps and other helper muscles. Taking a wide grip will increase the work on the lats, but from a strength training perspective you will likely be weaker. If looking to develop strength as the primary goal, keep your elbows in and increase the resistance. Additionally, when you keep your arms in, your improved leverage reduces the activity of the rear deltoids by using more middle trapezius help. Your choice of position should be based on your goal. If you are training for shape and look (overall appearance and functional strength), then you need to perform both variations; otherwise, decide which functional needs best suit you, and work through it.

Proper alignment is also very important. Keep your chest up and your head facing forward. Looking down or up will cause your back to round and involve other muscles in the lift, decreasing the overall contribution of the back muscles. Getting into a tight position—maintaining good posture, limiting extraneous movement, and keeping control—for any lift is essential. The back is no exception.

Remember that when working the upper back, the lower back must constantly support the movement. To perform exercises correctly, maintain proper back alignment. Stick your chest out, and keep your chin up—this will keep the lower back from rounding. Do not initiate upper back exercises with the lower back. Often lifters perform seated cable rows by leaning forward and jerking at the waist. This action prevents the lats and other back muscles from working through the entire range of motion. However, a bend at the waist to start, with a gentle leaning backward, may actually increase lat activation and also decrease the compressive load on the lower spine. Using the lower back and biceps to gain momentum during seated rows takes the work off the latissimus dorsi and decreases the rate of development.

When lifters have worked up to heavier weights, they may use straps to hold onto the bar. When lifting, grip strength in the forearms and hands usually fatigues before any other muscles. Straps present an attractive alternative to allow people to lift heavy. Many people say that straps relieve the grip muscle work and favor isolation of the lats, but generally they allow for a few more reps because they reduce the grip work. That sounds like a benefit, but if you increase your grip strength along with your back, you increase forearm strength and size as well as back strength. By allowing your grip strength to develop, you improve not only your overall pulling strength (which is more applicable for sport performance) but also your rate of progression. In some cases, straps allow the lifting of heavier weights but can also encourage bad form. Remember the principle of progression; you sacrifice form and development when you try to progress too quickly.

## — TRAIN AT HOME

### Pull Your Way to Stronger Lats

Hitting the lats is hard work and even harder without proper equipment. However, you can give yourself a great workout at home if you can find a way to do pull-ups or assisted pull-ups. The best option is to purchase a pull-up bar that attaches to a door frame (there are good ones now that are very sturdy). Another way to do pull-ups at home is by opening a door and fixing a rope (or belt or towel) around both doorknobs, leaving the rope ends free. Straddle the door with your legs, lay back at arm's length, grab the rope ends, and perform pull-ups as you would normally do by digging your heels into the floor and using them as the pivot point. For safety, be sure you can maintain a firm grip on the rope (or belt or towel) and that it is securely attached to the doorknobs.

Another method is to have a partner assist by standing over top of you while you are lying on the floor. (You should be lying between the partner's legs.) Grab your partner's hands or a towel your partner is holding, and pull yourself up so that your body pivots on your feet. Although the range of motion is short, it is better than nothing. If those methods do not appeal to you, then you can use resistance tubing in a manner similar to the pressing motions in chapter 5. Stand facing a pole of some kind, hook the middle of the tubing around the pole, and complete the pulling motions described in this chapter.

# BUILD YOUR BACK

Since the back is a critical body part, it should be exercised on its own as much as possible. Although you can't completely eliminate the biceps from back work, you can reduce their contribution by concentrating on using the back muscles to begin each movement. Move slowly and deliberately. Jerking the weight will activate the biceps first and may lead to grip fatigue.

One practical way to accomplish a complete back workout is to use a variety of pulls in your program. I recommend incorporating both the seated row and the lat pull-down into your workouts. A great way to target the back muscles from every angle is to perform fewer sets of each individual exercise but include more exercises. For a real challenge, try using the pullover in a pre- or postexhaust routine (see chapter 15 for more on pre- and postexhaustion) with the lat pull-down as shown in sample routine 3.

| Exercise | Number of sets | Reps per set | Rest between sets |
|---|---|---|---|
| **Routine 1** | | | |
| Bent-over barbell row | 3 | 8 | 2 min. |
| Straight-arm pull-down | 2 | 12 | 90 sec. |
| Front pull | 2 | 10 | 90 sec. |
| **Routine 2** | | | |
| Seated row | 3 | 10 | 90 sec. |
| Lat pull-down | 2 | 12 | 90 sec. |
| Dumbbell row | 2 | 8 | 90 sec. |
| **Routine 3** | | | |
| Lat pull-down | 3 | 12 | 90 sec. |
| Dumbbell pullover | 2 | 10 | 60 sec. |
| Reverse-grip bent-over barbell row | 2 | 8 | 90 sec. |

# 7

# SHOULDERS

The deltoids are actually three distinct muscles with three different functions. The anterior (front) deltoid raises your arm to the front of your body and pulls your arm across your body. The medial (middle) deltoid elevates your arm perpendicularly to your body (known as abduction) to move your arm out away from the side of your body. The posterior (rear) deltoid primarily pulls your arm back. The deltoids work in concert with the rotator cuff, a collective name that describes four small, deep muscles that hold the shoulders in place. These muscles allow the arm to rotate at the shoulder. When improper technique is used or the shoulder is overused, the muscles of the rotator cuff are often the ones that feel it.

Although many people love the idea of having boulders for shoulders, overworking these muscles can lead to problems. Remember, both the rotator cuff muscles and the deltoids will be worked during any upper body movement. The anterior deltoids work during pushing movements such as bench presses. The posterior deltoids work during pulling movements. The medial deltoids are worked in all exercises in which the arms are out away from your body in the abducted position. When trained properly, the deltoids can be both appealing and physically functional.

## Shoulder Press

The king of shoulder exercises is certainly the shoulder press, also known as the military press. This exercise can be performed using dumbbells, a barbell, or a machine.

1. Sit on a weight bench, holding a dumbbell in each hand. Lift the dumbbells to your shoulders, palms facing forward, elbows in line with your shoulders.
2. Push the weights up until your arms are fully extended.
3. Gently lock your elbows. Pause for two counts at the top of the motion. Keep your torso tight and your chest and chin up during this exercise.
4. Return the weights to the starting position at your shoulders. Resist the momentum as the weights descend.

Overtraining the shoulders is the most common symptom of using too much weight too quickly. It is better to underdo it than to overdo it. Do not compromise your lower back in order to use more weight. Do not use momentum or bounce the weight during the movement.

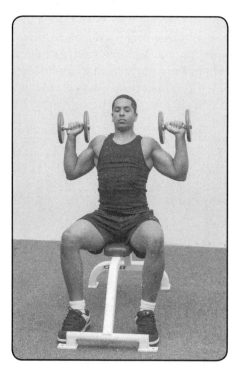

Starting position

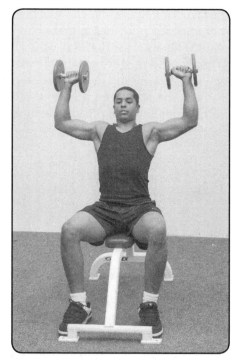

Push weights up

A great way to isolate shoulders so your weaker side can catch up is to perform alternating single-arm dumbbell presses. By alternating pressing movements and keeping the dumbbell under constant tension, the body continually rights itself, improving both the size and shape of the deltoid while forcing the rest of the body to develop strength in the support and balance muscles. When you perform the single-arm version, be sure each rep is individual and deliberate. Although tempting, do not get into a bicycling type of pattern. If you use a bar, you can lower it behind or in front of your head. Beginners should keep the bar in front to reduce neck strain on the cervical disc area and to prevent possible shoulder impingement. Once you have good technique and range of motion (and as long as you have no shoulder problems), you can lower the weight behind your head. The more posterior the bar or dumbbells travel, the greater the emphasis on the middle (medial) deltoid muscles.

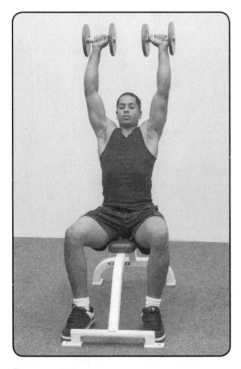

Pause at top

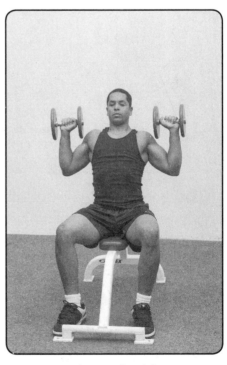

Return weights to shoulders

## Barbell Shoulder Press

The barbell shoulder press can be performed while sitting on a weight bench or while standing, although the sitting position is recommended for beginners.

1. Hold the bar with your hands slightly more than shoulder-width apart so that the bar touches the top of your chest.
2. Push the bar overhead, fully extending your arms. Lean back only far enough to allow the bar to pass in front of your head.
3. Once at the top, pause for two counts, then lower the bar back down under control. Oh, and watch your head—it may get in the way. (You also can start this exercise with your arms fully extended, lowering the weight to your chest as the first movement.)

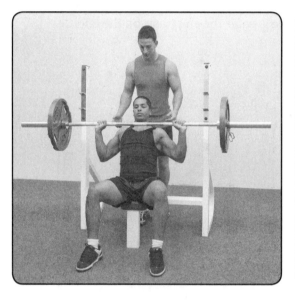 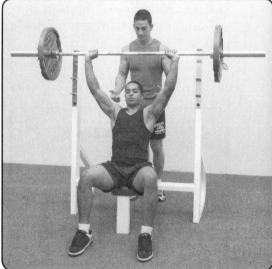

# Front Raise

The front raise targets the anterior deltoid.

1. Sit on a weight bench, arms at your sides, hands holding the dumbbells slightly to the front of your body. Your palms should be facing back.
2. Raise the dumbbells straight out in front of you until your arms are about shoulder height.
3. Lower the dumbbells back to the starting position. You also can perform this exercise with a barbell. Using an incline bench increases the range of motion. For greater range of motion, use an incline bench and lean back against it to lengthen the distance the dumbbell has to travel.

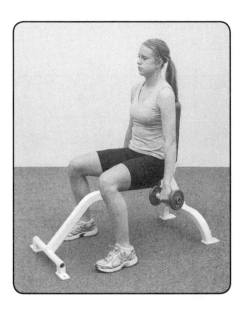 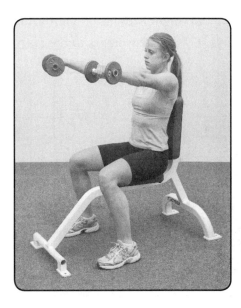

## Lateral Raise

The lateral raise, also called the side raise, isolates the medial deltoid. You can perform this exercise sitting on a weight bench (as shown) or standing. Standing requires a little more discipline and technique to maintain good posture and eliminate the tendency to cheat by throwing the weight up using the legs rather than forcing the shoulders to do their job. Experienced lifters can use either technique, but if you are just starting out, the seated position will force tighter form and isolate the deltoid muscles better.

1. Sit comfortably on the bench with your chest and head up. Grab a pair of dumbbells and hold them at your sides with your arms fully extended. Turn your palms toward you.
2. Raise your arms laterally until they are parallel with the ground, forming 90-degree angles at your armpits. Keep your elbows slightly bent.
3. Lower the weights to the starting position.

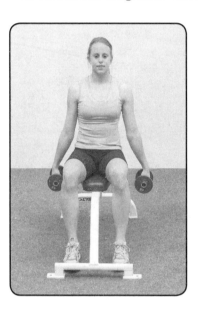
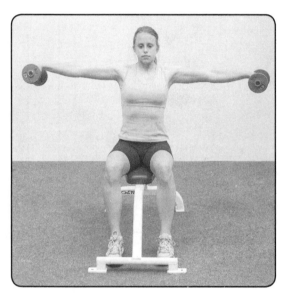

# Rear Deltoid Fly

The rear deltoid fly works the posterior deltoid and requires a little more patience. Start with a set of dumbbells resting on the floor on either side of the end of a bench.

1. Sit at the end of the bench and lean forward so that your upper back is parallel with the floor and your chest meets your knees. Keep your head in line with your back by looking at the floor. Drop your arms straight down, and grab the dumbbells with your palms facing each other.

2. Raise your arms to the sides and away from your body until they are parallel with the floor. Keep your elbows slightly bent.

3. Pause for two counts at the top of the movement, then return the weights to the floor. Try to keep the weights suspended from the floor between reps to keep the tension on the muscles the entire time.

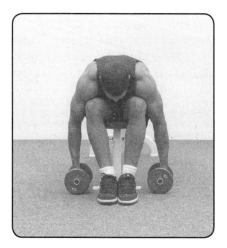 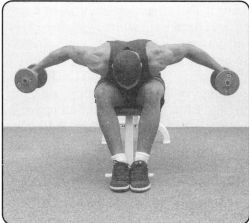

## — TAKE IT TO THE GYM

### Deltoids: Boulders for Shoulders

For men, broad shoulders may be a defining measure of manliness. For women, well-defined shoulders may provide better posture and confidence. Focusing on these hard-to-work muscles is the key to developing size. However, be careful not to overtrain. The most important concept to remember is that less is better than more. Since these muscles are used during almost every upper body exercise, often one or two sets of isolated shoulder work are plenty when mixed with other exercises. If you train your shoulders on their own, be sure to allow adequate rest between workouts. Try to use dumbbells as much as possible. Dumbbells not only develop your ability to stabilize and balance the weight, strengthening the rotator cuff, but also provide a greater range of motion.

Working the shoulder muscles can lead to back problems if you aren't cautious. Contract your abdominal muscles during the movement, and keep your head and chest up. Use lighter weights, and make your movements more defined. Do not use momentum to move the weights. Dropping your body to help lift the weight will only decrease the shoulder muscle involvement. Since safety is of the utmost concern, using perfect form and minimizing lower back involvement are imperative. The most common error in weight training is to allow the body to bend and the lower back to round.

Gravity may be your worst enemy in performing overhead lifts. More than one lifter has gotten a good headache while performing shoulder presses, so be sure to clear your head. If you begin to feel yourself failing during the lift, lower the weight. Continuing after failure can do serious damage to the shoulder capsule.

## — TRAIN AT HOME

### Train Your Shoulder Boulders at Home

If you are a little older, you may remember the days when you or your brother could do push-ups standing on your head. If you have a no-fear approach and have considerable strength, shoulder pressing your weight while inverted against a wall for support is a great exercise, but be careful since this approach requires some balance and flexibility. For the rest of you mere mortals, try doing shoulder presses with resistance tubing. Standing on the middle of the tubing (or fixing it under a chair if you are sitting) and pressing the handles from shoulder height up will give you a good workout. You can take that same position and lighten the bands for both front and side raises. To get to your rear delts, you can use the rear deltoid fly and complete a reverse fly by pulling your arms backward while they are fully extended and perpendicular to your body. The scarecrow row (see chapter 8) will also target your rear deltoids.

# DIG THOSE DELTS

If you are prepared to work out more than three times a week, these shoulder routines will give you a good challenge. Routines 2 and 3 show a sample posterior and anterior combination routine for chest and back days.

| Exercise | Number of sets | Reps per set | Rest between sets |
|---|---|---|---|
| **Routine 1** | | | |
| Dumbbell shoulder press | 3 | 8 | 2 min. |
| Front raise | 2 | 10 | 60 sec. |
| Rear deltoid fly | 2 | 12 | 60 sec. |
| **Routine 2** | | | |
| Barbell shoulder press | 3 | 10 | 2 min. |
| Rear deltoid fly | 3 | 10 | 90 sec. |
| Front raise | 2 | 10 | 90 sec. |
| **Routine 3** | | | |
| Single-arm dumbbell press* | 2 | 12 | 90 sec. |
| Lateral raise | 3 | 12 | 90 sec. |
| Rear deltoid fly | 3 | 12 | 60 sec. |

*Refer to page 79 for more about performing the single-arm dumbbell press.

# 8

# TRAPS

A hallmark of bodybuilding success is to have traps, or trapezius muscles, that touch the ears, although your aspirations may not be as high. There are three distinct parts of the trapezius, classified by location. The upper portion, the one most people are familiar with, helps you perform shoulder elevations (e.g., when you shrug your shoulders). The middle portion helps stabilize the scapulae and also aids in pulling your arms in by performing scapular retraction (squeezing your shoulder blades together). The bottom portion helps in depressing the shoulder blades, which is generally not a common function. However, if you've ever spent too much time in front of a computer and your shoulders started hunching up, you may have used your lower traps to pull your shoulders down to stretch the neck and upper trap. The lower trap is also what allows you to keep your arms at your sides if you happen to be hanging upside down.

The traps are responsible for maintaining proper posture of the middle and upper back, the neck, and the shoulder blades. The traps are also important for reducing long-term injury. Don't be afraid to do trap work for fear of looking like a Neanderthal. In fact you stand a better chance of not looking like one if you work your traps. Increasing the strength of the upper back, scapulae, and neck muscles keeps tight posture and may reduce some of the "hunching over" (kyphosis) that sometimes occurs later in life. Working the traps can help maintain function and independence down the road.

The traps also help you perform the upper back exercises in chapter 6. Traps aid in pulling motions and help pull the shoulder blades together. The traps rarely function alone, so isolating them is difficult. However, there are a few neat ways to target these muscles.

# Shoulder Shrug

The shoulder shrug is definitely the most popular and easy to execute trapezius exercise. You can execute the exercise with either a barbell or dumbbells. The key to successful performance is tight form and relying on the traps to do the work. Avoid using your legs to initiate the movement.

1. To perform shoulder shrugs with a barbell, stand with feet about shoulder-width apart, knees gently locked. Hold the barbell at arm's length down in front of you with your hands about shoulder-width apart, palms turned toward you. (You also can perform this exercise while holding the barbell behind your back.)

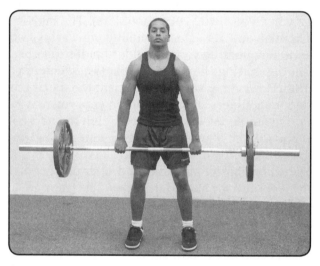

Starting position

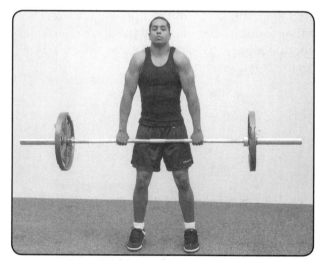

Lift your shoulders

2. Lift your shoulders, squeezing your traps up toward your ears.
3. Pause for two counts at the top, then lower the bar back to the starting position.

To perform shoulder shrugs with dumbbells, stand with feet about shoulder-width apart, knees gently locked. Hold one dumbbell in each hand at your sides with your palms turned toward you. Lift your shoulders, squeezing your traps. Pause for two counts at the top of the movement, then return the weights to the starting position.

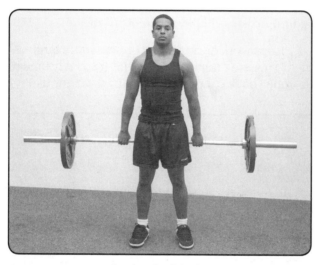

Starting position for barbell behind back

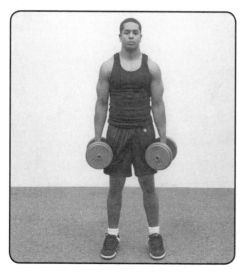

Starting position with dumbbells

## Upright Row

The main trap exercise besides the shoulder shrug is the upright row. The upright row primarily works the traps, but they get a lot of help from the medial deltoids. Because the upright row puts pressure on the shoulder capsule, do not perform this exercise if you have shoulder problems.

1. Stand with feet shoulder-width apart, knees slightly bent. Hold the barbell in front, palms turned toward you.
2. Pull the barbell straight up, shooting your elbows out to the sides. The bar should follow along your ribs until it hits the top of your chest.
3. Pause for two counts at the top of the movement, and shrug before slowly lowering the bar back to the starting point. Do not begin the motion by shrugging first or you will place the brunt of the load on the deltoids.

Remember, the traps work during many upper back exercises. The shoulder shrug and upright row are enough to give the traps a little extra work when combined with upper back exercises in a sound weight training program.

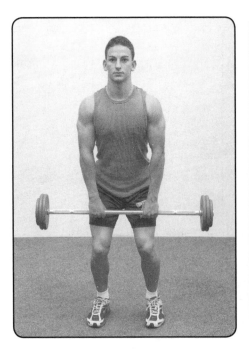 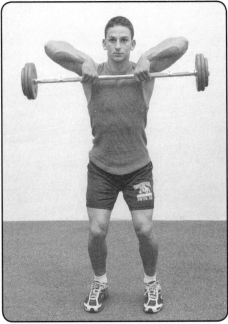

## Scarecrow Row

Trapezius isolation is difficult; however, a great way to get the rear delts fired up along with your traps is this move that takes its name from the body position used to perform it.

1. Affix the middle of a piece of resistance tubing around a solid object or pole, and stand facing it while grabbing the handles in either hand. (This exercise can be performed with a pulley machine using separate handles attached to the same pulley by chains.) Raise your arms up in front, forming a 90-degree angle at your armpits so that your arms are parallel with the ground. Turn your palms toward each other, and step back so that the tubing is taut.
2. Keeping your arms fully extended, squeeze your shoulder blades together, and pull your hands apart and arms back and out to your sides so that you form a T with your body. This is the scarecrow position.
3. Hold for two counts before returning to the starting position.

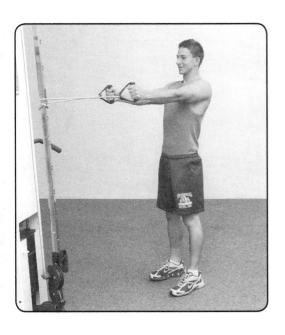 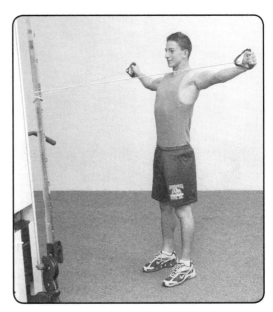

## Scapular Retraction

This exercise is a great way to target your middle trapezius muscle, and although the range of motion is very short, scapular retraction is both therapeutic and effective.

1. Face a cable machine either standing or seated. Using a straight bar attachment at chest height, fully extend your arms and take an overhand grip. Take up the slack by positioning your body so that your arms are locked out front and the cable is taut.

2. Keeping the arms locked while fully extended, squeeze your shoulder blades together. Hold for two counts, then release your blades all the way open so that the resistance pulls your arms out, rounding your upper back as much as possible. Again, don't let this short range of motion fool you; this is a good exercise, especially if you have shoulder instability.

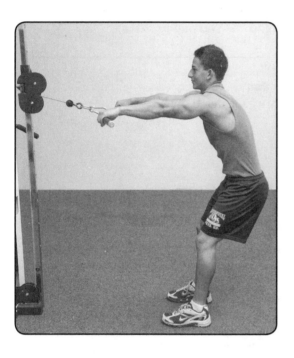 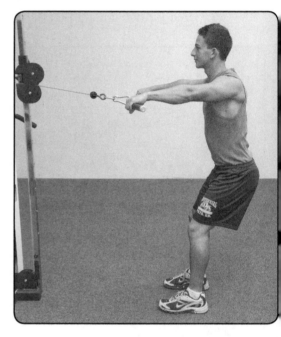

## — TAKE IT TO THE GYM

### Focus on the Motion

As you execute shoulder shrugs, think about the movement you make when indicating "I don't know" to work on isolating the trapezius muscles. The motion is exactly the same. Remember to pull your traps to your ears and squeeze tightly. You can also try verbalizing when you get to the top of the movement to increase your motivation.

If you lift heavy weights, you can use straps to hold onto the bar, particularly if your grip strength is weak. In this case, straps may be necessary since your traps can handle quite a bit of weight and often a lot more than your wrists can. Remember, though, that straps impede your development of grip strength, so if your grip strength can handle heavy enough weights to wear your traps down without using straps, then do not get in the practice of using them. In addition, avoid using your legs when you lift. Use of momentum will prevent proper development of the traps. Control the execution of the movement, pausing for two counts to allow the traps to develop, decrease the contribution of the deltoids, and prevent strain of the rotator cuff.

Many so-called experts will tell you to roll your shoulders forward and back at the top of the lift. This is not necessary and will not increase the emphasis on the traps. Worse yet, it may put the shoulder in a bad position. Although they are uncommon, shoulder dislocations have occurred when lifters tried to roll the shoulders.

## — TRAIN AT HOME

### Home-Based Trap Development

Mechanically speaking, your traps are in a good position to lift quite a bit of weight. Whether you are strength training or looking for shape or endurance, performing shoulder shrugs at home is both easy and recommended. The same exercise you would perform with a barbell or dumbbells can be done with resistance tubing. If you are standing, grab the handles and hold the middle of the tubing to the ground with your foot. Perform the same shrugs, pulling straight up with your shoulders and keeping your arms locked at full length. To perform the exercise seated, you can lock the tubing around your feet out in front, maintain an erect or slightly backward leaning position, and perform the same shrugging motion by pulling on the handles.

# TRAINING THE TRAPS

Trapezius variations are not very complex, but keeping things simple is often more desirable. The mini routines will address the needs of your training program and help maintain proper posture. Often trap work is performed on the same day as shoulder work (e.g., rear deltoid fly).

| Exercise | Number of sets | Reps per set | Rest between sets |
|---|---|---|---|
| **Routine 1** | | | |
| Shoulder shrug | 3 | 10 | 90 sec. |
| Scapular retraction | 3 | 12 | 60 sec. |
| Upright row | 2 | 8 | 90 sec. |
| **Routine 2** | | | |
| Upright row | 3 | 8 | 90 sec. |
| Shoulder shrug | 3 | 8 | 90 sec. |
| Rear deltoid fly | 2 | 12 | 60 sec. |
| **Routine 3** | | | |
| Scapular retraction | 2 | 15 | 60 sec. |
| Upright row | 2 | 15 | 90 sec. |
| Shoulder shrug | 2 | 10 | 90 sec. |
| Rear deltoid fly | 2 | 10 | 60 sec. |

# 9

# ARMS

Because your arms are involved in virtually every task you do on a daily basis, having a little extra arm strength and endurance is an asset that nobody can argue. Often look and shape is the main reason young men train their arms, but vanity alone is not the only reason to target them for men or women. In a relatively short time, with a few simple exercises, you will get that nice shape. If size is not your thing, don't worry; increasing bulk takes considerably longer and requires discipline and training volume.

Your arms are composed of the larger triceps muscle group in the back, the biceps muscles in the front, and your forearms. The triceps muscle group is responsible for extending the arm at the elbow. The triceps is involved in many throwing and pushing activities. As the name implies, the triceps muscle has three heads, all similar in function. While there is evidence that each muscle head can be trained individually with specific exercises, most research indicates that genetics rather than training may be responsible for any differences. For beginners, focus on good execution of all extension exercises. A common goal is to make this muscle have a horseshoe-like appearance when it is contracted.

The biceps are the most flexed and visible muscles of the body. In many cases, the biceps are the focal point of a lifter's routine. Interestingly, this two-headed muscle is not the only one that flexes the arm. Two other strong flexors, the brachialis and brachioradialis, work when you target this area. Contrary to popular belief, no single exercise can develop the biceps' specific shape. Hard work and some help from genetics are necessary.

The forearms contain many muscles that flex the wrist and fingers. Eating spinach has been shown to increase forearm size in some cartoon characters, but most people need to perform gripping-type exercises to see improvements. The forearms get a lot of work during many pulling exercises if done without using lifting straps.

# Dumbbell Curl

The easiest biceps exercise to perform is also one of the best ways to target the biceps. The dumbbell curl can be performed sitting or standing, alternating arms or moving both together.

1. Stand with your arms fully extended down at your sides. Grab the dumbbells with your hands semipronated (palms facing toward each other), with your thumbs facing forward.

2. Slowly begin to flex your arms by contracting your biceps. The dumbbells should follow an arc as the angle at your elbows decreases. Your elbows should be fixed at your sides during the entire movement.

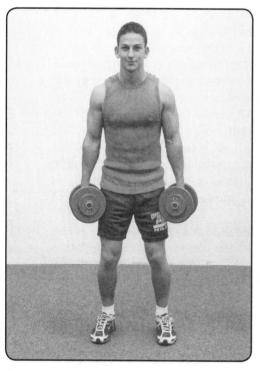

Starting position

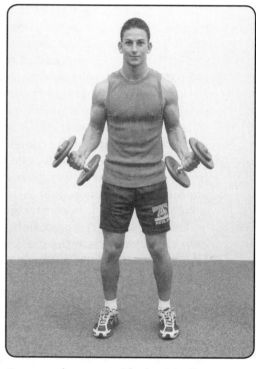

Contract biceps to lift dumbbells

3. Bring the dumbbells to your shoulders, and squeeze your biceps tight for two counts. During the movement, twist the dumbbells so your palms face toward your shoulders to maximally activate the biceps. Slowly lower the dumbbells back to your sides.

Keeping your hands semipronated during the movement will focus more on the brachioradialis, giving the front of the lower arm more of a challenge. Supinating (turning the wrists out) on the way up has been shown to activate the biceps more fully, so for big biceps training, turn your palms up and out as you come up.

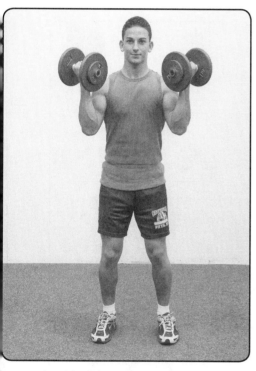

Bring dumbbells to shoulders

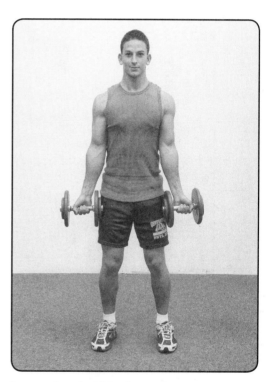

Lower the dumbbells

# Triceps Push-Down

The triceps can be worked in several ways. One of the easiest and most effective ways is to use a cable machine to perform the triceps push-down. This exercise may have its own station in the gym, or you can use the lat pull-down area. Select a bar attachment that is comfortable for your grip. Although many lifters think different types of bars hit the triceps differently, most research says otherwise.

1. Stand and grab the bar with your hands at chest height and with the palms facing forward. Your arms should be fully flexed, with your elbows against your sides. Your hands should be approximately shoulder-width apart. (If you use an inverted-V bar, your hands will be slightly closer.)

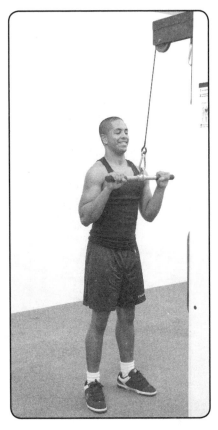

Starting position

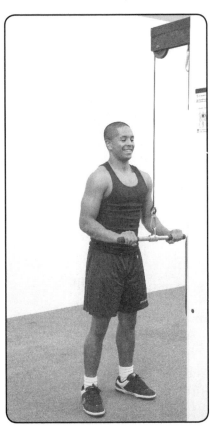

Press arms down

2. Lock your elbows at your sides, and press the bar down until your arms are fully extended. The motion should be in a single plane. Keep your elbows in during the entire movement.

3. At the bottom position, squeeze your triceps.

4. Slowly return the bar to the starting position. Some lifters return the bar only to about waist height before beginning the next rep, but you want to use as large a range of motion as possible, so bring the bar all the way back up to chest height. Before you begin the next rep, your elbow angle should be as small as possible.

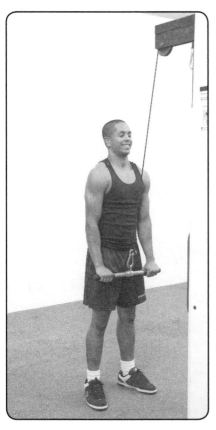

Squeeze triceps at bottom

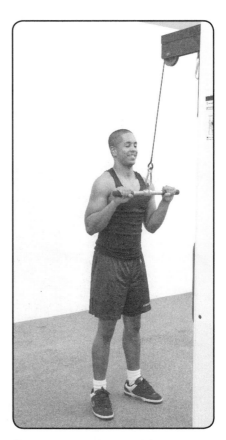

Return to starting position

# Wrist Curl

This easy exercise works both sides of the arm. You can use either dumbbells or a barbell; however, the barbell's length makes it more difficult to manipulate. You can work one arm at a time or both arms simultaneously.

1. Kneel next to a chair or weight bench with your forearms resting on the chair or bench and your wrists hanging over the edge.
2. To work the flexors on the inside of the arms, rest the outsides of your forearms on the chair or bench. Grab the dumbbells with your palms facing up. Slowly raise and lower the dumbbells by flexing and releasing your wrists. Make each movement deliberate, and go through the full range of motion.

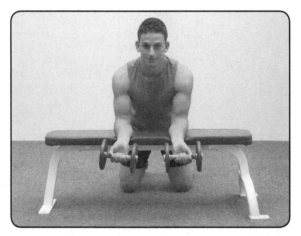

Starting position to work flexors

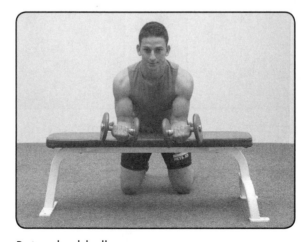

Raise dumbbells

3. To work the extensors on the back side of your arms, rest the insides of your forearms on the chair or bench. Grab the dumbbells with your palms facing down. Slowly raise and lower the dumbbells by flexing and releasing your wrists.

The variety of exercises that work this muscle group is rather meager. One variation that works your grip is hanging wrist work. Grab very large dumbbells and hold them at your sides for as long as you can. Another variation is to use a slightly lighter dumbbell and roll it to the ends of your fingers and back up. In other words, open your hand until the weight reaches the ends of your fingers, then curl your fingers and roll the dumbbell back into your palm. Perform this exercise with extreme caution; if you drop the weight, your toes may never forgive you. A third variation is to buy a set of grippers. Hold the grippers in your hands and squeeze them tightly.

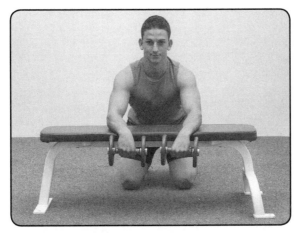

Starting position to work extensors

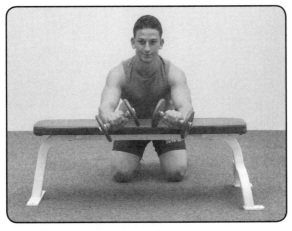

Raise dumbbells

## Isolated Dumbbell Curl

In the isolated dumbbell curl, one arm is worked at a time.

1. Sit on a weight bench. Press the back of your working arm against your inner thigh. Begin with the dumbbell in your hand, your arm fully extended.
2. Slowly flex your arm, lifting the weight to your shoulder.
3. Pause at the top of the movement, and squeeze your biceps. Return the weight to the starting position.

For variation, turn your palm inward as if you were holding a hammer, and follow the same curling motion, keeping your lower arm in this position throughout the movement. This curl targets the brachioradialis slightly more and is known as the hammer curl.

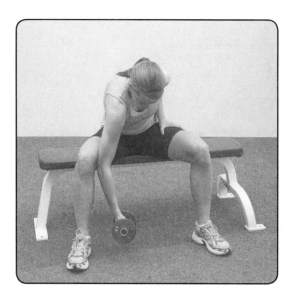 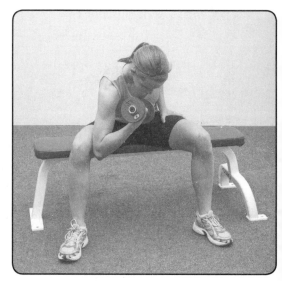

## Straight Bar Curl

Probably the most common curl is the standing curl, also known as the straight bar curl. This exercise can be done with a standard straight barbell (straight bar curl) or a cambered E-Z bar (standing curl). Avoid lower back injuries by making the biceps work harder—don't lean back.

1. Stand behind the barbell. Lock your hands around the bar, palms up, hands spread a little more than shoulder-width apart. Stand holding the barbell, arms fully extended.
2. Slowly raise the barbell to your shoulders. The weight follows an arc until the arms are fully flexed.
3. Lower the bar to the starting position under control; it should take about 3 to 4 seconds to lower it.

For variation, start with your hands spread wider on the bar, six inches (15 cm) or so from your body.

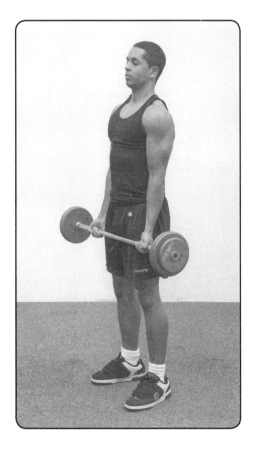 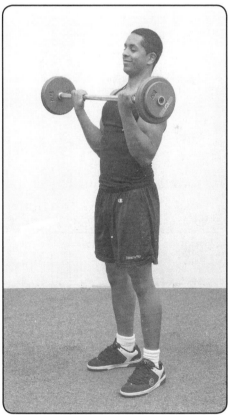

# Cable Curl

The cable curl can also be done using a single handle fixed to a low pulley position on a machine.

1. Grab the handle with both hands, and pull it up to the extended-arm starting position. Force yourself to keep your elbows in at your sides.
2. Slowly flex your arms, raising the handle to your shoulders.
3. Squeeze your biceps at the top of the movement. Slowly return to the starting position.

For variation, use a single handle and try the hammer curl position (see page 102).

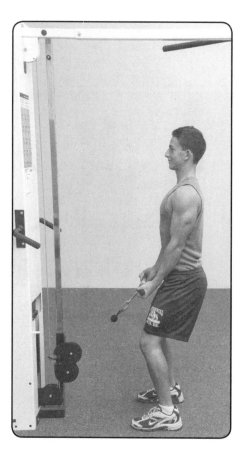 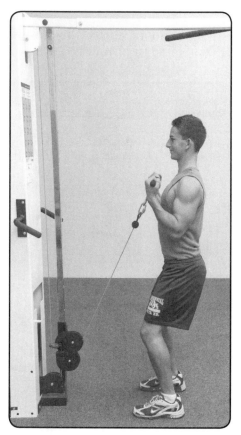

# Preacher Curl

The preacher curl makes a great isolated movement and can be performed using a preacher bench or with a machine. This exercise does a good job of isolating the arm by fixing it and preventing cheating by using other muscles. If you use a preacher bench, you can use either a cambered E-Z bar or a straight bar. If you use a machine, make sure your elbows are lined up properly with the machine.

1. If you use the preacher bench, lean over the bench, fixing your armpits tightly to the bench. For a machine, grab the handles on the machine, palms up, arms extended.
2. Slowly flex your arms, bringing the handles or bar to your shoulders.
3. Pause for two counts at the top of the movement, and squeeze your biceps. Slowly return to the starting position.

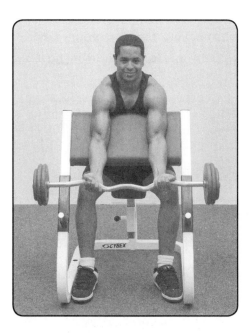 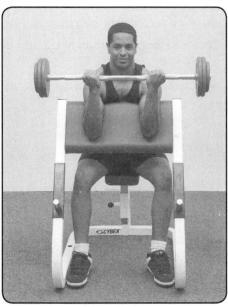

# Reverse-Grip Barbell Curl

Although targeting the biceps is best done in isolation with a supinated (palms up) grip, reversing your hands so that your palms face down (pronated grip) requires you to grip harder to keep the weight from falling out of your hands. This works the brachialis slightly more as well as incorporates a little more help from wrist flexor muscles. The motion in reverse-grip curling is the same as when standing or seated at a preacher bench. The range of motion is slightly short, and learning to grip and hold the bar takes a little getting used to at first. You can select either a straight bar or E-Z curl bar based on your comfort. If you are short on time and want to kill two birds with one stone, this is a good choice for your biceps and forearms.

1. Grab the bar with an overhand grip so that your palms are facing down. Take a slightly wider than shoulder-width stance, with a slight bend in your knees.
2. Lift the bar so it's across the tops of your thighs, and fix your elbows tight to your body.
3. Flex your arms, bringing the barbell from your thighs to your chest.
4. Hold for two counts at the top before returning to your starting position at your thighs.

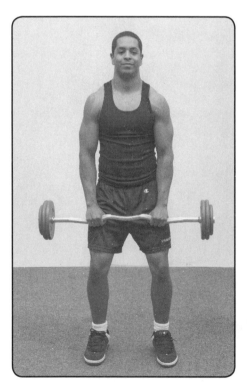 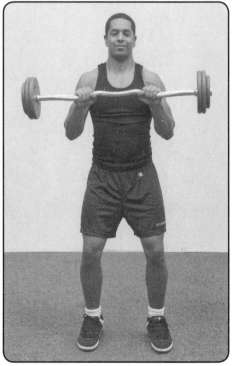

## Supine Triceps Extension

The supine triceps extension, also known as the skull crusher, nose breaker, or head caver, targets the triceps effectively when performed properly. You can use a barbell or dumbbells for this exercise. If one is available, consider using a cambered bar because it is more comfortable to grip.

1. Lie on your back on a weight bench. Grab the bar, and bring it to a position just behind your head. Your elbows should point straight forward and up. The angle at the armpits should be just past 90 or up to 120 degrees. Your palms should be up.

2. Fully extend your arms. When your arms are fully extended, the weight should be over your chin, not over your eyes. Keeping the arms in proper position keeps the tension on the triceps.

3. Hold for two counts at this fully contracted position before returning to the starting position just behind your head. Some people prefer to bring the weight to their foreheads (hence the name skull crusher), but for both safety and longer range of motion, behind the head is your better choice.

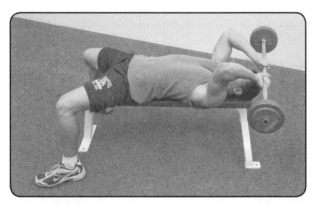

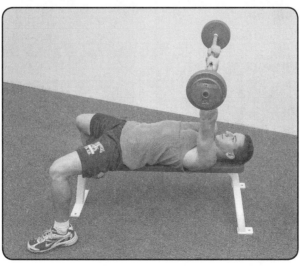

## Dip

The dip is definitely the king of triceps exercises. Dips also work the chest and front deltoids. To do dips, you need to have plenty of strength and balance. The great thing about doing dips is that you use your own body weight. If you can't complete a full set of dips, then do as many as you can. In time, you will be amazed at how easy they are.

1. Hoist yourself onto the parallel bars with your body between them. Start with your arms fully extended by your sides.
2. Bend your elbows, slowly lowering yourself between the bars until your elbows form a 90-degree angle.
3. Pause for two counts, then return to the starting position by pushing down against the bars.

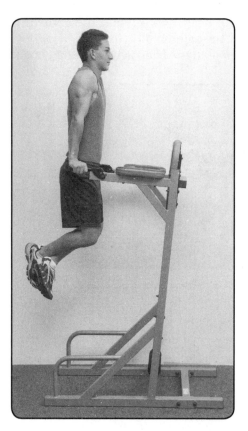 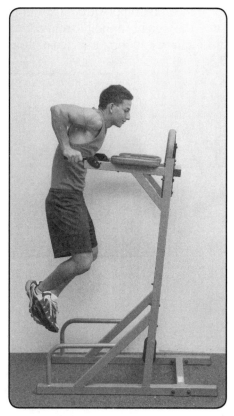

# Bench Dip

If you have trouble performing dips on parallel bars, the modified bench dip is a good alternative.

1. Begin with your feet on a flat bench and your legs fully extended. Your arms should be shoulder-width apart with your hands on the bench directly behind you, fingertips facing forward. This is a slightly awkward position, and you will feel a stretch across your chest.

2. Bend your elbows, slowly lowering your body until your elbows form a 90-degree angle.

3. Pause for two counts, then return to the starting position by pushing your arms downward.

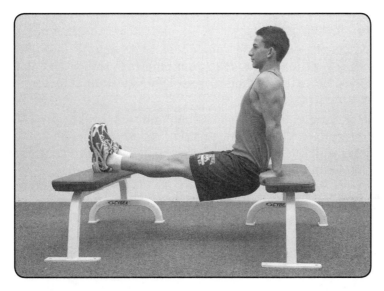

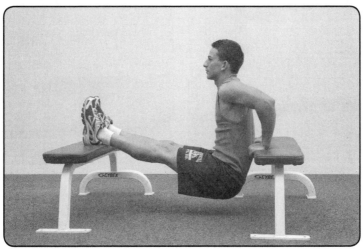

## Close-Grip Bench Press

Although we discuss chest training in chapter 5, getting a little help from the pecs may be just the added edge that your triceps need. The close-grip version of a bench press does not completely isolate the triceps but does a very good job at making them the primary target when your hands are positioned close to each other.

1. Using the same form as for your regular bench press, move your hands in closer together. Traditional wide-grip bench pressers (such as powerlifters and strongmen) find that a shoulder-width grip is close enough. Others may want to use a grip that is about 6 inches (15 cm) apart. Some lifters bring their hands together so that they are touching, but this position may be too stressful for some.

2. Take the bar from the rack as you would for a regular bench press. Make sure your body is tight.

3. Inhale deeply, expanding your chest, and begin to lower the weight. As you lower the weight, keep your elbows in rather than flared out to the sides. Bring the barbell closer to your sternum than for the regular bench press.

4. Pause at your chest for two counts, and then press upward, exhaling and returning to the starting position. As you are pressing, concentrate on using your triceps, and keep your elbows tight to your chest rather than flared out to the sides.

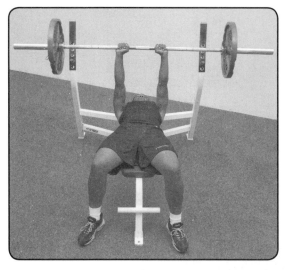 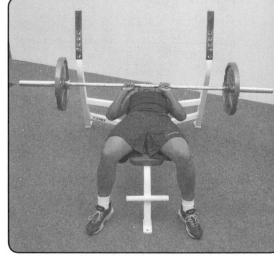

## Dumbbell Triceps Kickback

Another popular exercise is the dumbbell triceps kickback. In this exercise, you work one arm at a time. Keep your elbow high throughout the movement.

1. Stand with feet about shoulder-width apart, knees slightly bent. Lean forward and place your nonlifting hand on a knee for support. Maintain a flat back. Grasp the dumbbell firmly in your lifting hand. Point your elbow toward the ceiling.

2. Extend your lifting arm back as far as comfortable. Full extension should feel slightly uncomfortable; if it doesn't, your elbow may not be high enough.

3. Pause for two counts at the top, then return to the starting position.

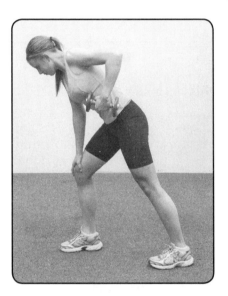 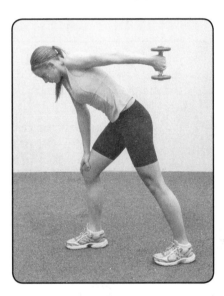

# Overhead Triceps Extension

A variation of the dumbbell triceps kickback is to perform the same movement overhead.

1. Stand with feet shoulder-width apart, or sit on a weight bench. Keep your back flat. Hold the dumbbell in one hand. Bring your lifting elbow up next to your ear.

2. Point your elbow toward the ceiling. Fully extend your arm. The dumbbell will travel behind your head to the overhead position.

3. Pause for two counts at the top before slowly lowering the bar back behind your head to the starting position. Don't rush here. You may want to move your head slightly forward or to the side to avoid an ugly collision!

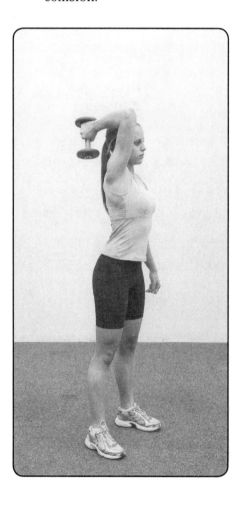 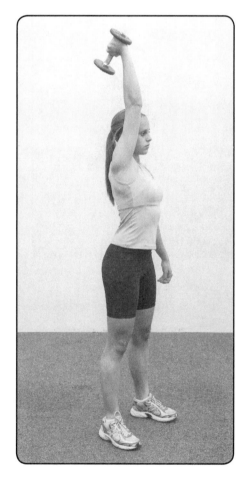

# Cable Reverse-Grip Triceps Pull-Down

Although not a common exercise, this variation of the triceps push-down can be performed with one arm at a time or with both arms together. Use either a handle (for single arm) or a straight or bent bar attachment (for both arms) on the same cable triceps push-down machine. At first, you will need lighter weight because this exercise will feel a little funny as you get used to the grip, but you should feel your triceps working over time to get the weight moving.

1. Face the pulley stack, keep your elbow in tight to your sides, and use a reverse grip (palms up), starting with the handle at chest height.
2. Pull the bar down, extending your arm fully.
3. Pause at the fully extended position, and then return to the start.

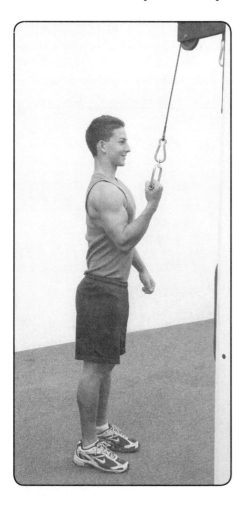
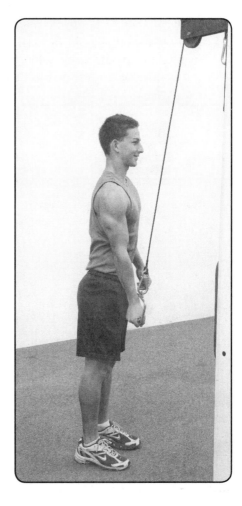

# Wrist Roller

A great way to hit just about all of the wrist muscles is to "roll" them out. These can be done anywhere, and although there are specific devices to do this movement, you can make a wrist roller quite easily. To make your own, you need some rope and a dowel, broomstick, or even PVC tubing. Make the dowel, which becomes the handle or bar, about 12 inches (30 cm) long. Tie one end of a rope around the middle of the dowel. Let the rest of the rope hang down, and tie the other end around a dumbbell or through the hole of an Olympic plate.

1. Grab the dowel with a hand on either side of the rope. Extend your arms out in front of you, maintaining a slight bend at the elbows.
2. Alternate hand action to create a rolling action on the bar so that the rope rolls onto the dowel. Keep going until the weight meets the dowel.
3. Roll the rope back out (and the weight down) slowly and under control using the opposite motion. Increase the resistance so that it is difficult but not impossible to get the weight up to the top and back without fatiguing.

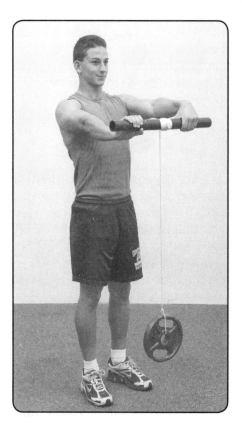 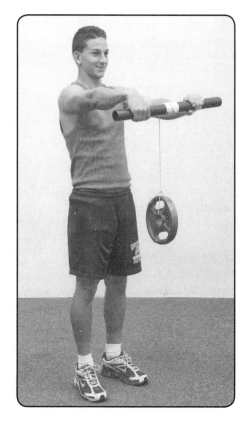

# TAKE IT TO THE GYM

## Building Better Biceps

A trick for standing exercises is to bend your legs slightly, taking pressure off your lower back, and stagger your feet to create more balance. As the weight gets farther from your body during the movement, you will need more force to overcome its relative weight. You need good balance and control.

One of the biggest mistakes lifters make is to start the movement by launching the bar or dumbbell with momentum. Creating momentum at the waist causes the lifter to lean back, moving the tension from the biceps to other muscle groups. Lifters often cheat at biceps exercises when it gets most difficult, usually at the 90-degree angle. However, working through that sticking point will truly enhance overall improvement in the biceps. The desire to cheat by launching the weight with momentum is natural, but the best results will come if you force yourself to work harder when it gets harder.

Developing the biceps takes time and patience. Don't give up on them. Any pulling exercise will work these muscles. If you are having a difficult time developing these muscles, try isolating your arm muscles by inserting an arm-only day into your training program once a week. No single exercise can effectively target a specific area of the biceps, so your keys to success are performing a variety of exercises and using a full range of motion.

Another good tip is to get a spotter to assist you. Don't be afraid to get some help. Instead of using momentum and cheating through the tough areas, get a buddy to help you a little, and force your body to remain upright during the lift. To really work your biceps, try 10 reps with a heavy weight, forcing the last few reps.

## Tips to Tone Triceps

Proper execution is the key to success. During triceps exercises, the less you move your elbow back and forth, the more you emphasize the triceps. Maintaining proper posture is a must. To keep proper posture, contract your abs and keep your chest up. Many lifters note that the abs feel as if they work during triceps exercises. This is a good thing because it means that proper body posture is being used.

To get a true horseshoe-like appearance in your triceps, use the entire range of motion. That means using a smaller dumbbell and lighter weights. When you extend your arms, use a gentle lock at your elbows; do not snap them into a full lockout. Use a thumb-lock grip. A loose grip will prevent overexertion, but you need to be able to hold onto the barbell or dumbbell. The most important tip, however, is to make sure that the plates are secured to the barbell or dumbbell. You will quickly learn why supine triceps extensions are called nose breakers if a plate falls off while you are performing one.

Although injuries are rare, olecranon bursitis (swelling in the elbow) may occur if you overdo it. If your elbow is sore, do not do triceps exercises. If you feel a slight pain during a particular exercise, try a different hand grip. It is not uncommon to find that some exercises bother the elbow but others don't.

## Get a Grip!

Do not neglect grip work in your training, especially if you play tennis, golf, baseball, softball, or any other sport that requires you to hold a hitting implement. The heavier the weight you use and the slower you perform the movement, the greater the training effect will be.

Using dumbbells with spinning plates allows the weight to move properly, but if you don't have dumbbells with spinning plates, don't worry. For the most part, if the dumbbell plates are secure, then wrist curls are safe. It is difficult to do any major damage unless you really overwork your wrists. The first few times you do these exercises, you may get sore, but in time the soreness will go away and your grip strength will improve dramatically.

# — TRAIN AT HOME —

## Home-Based Pipe Training

For those of you looking to get in shape, you have several options for working out your arms at home. If you are looking for a quick pump, you can get that swollen look without the gym. If you take a good look around, you'll discover a variety of home training tools, and when you understand the way a muscle is worked, you can find a method to stress them enough to create a challenge.

Using the straight bar curl position, you can curl resistance tubing to work your biceps. The best way to make use of the tubing is to grab the handles on either side and stand on the middle. For your triceps, pull the tubing up to your shoulders, extend your elbows overhead, and perform arm extensions overhead (triceps extensions). Don't forget about your own body weight. Doing push-ups with your hands together will get a good triceps burn. There are also plenty of heavy objects in your house that you can curl. Grab either end of a rolled towel with someone else or an object hanging from the middle. Pull upward on the towel handles, creating a curl-like movement for the biceps.

Training your forearms at home is also an easy task. If you have made your own wrist roller you are set, but another option is to grab nearly any object in your house that is heavy enough to make your forearms work. Popular items include soup cans, heavy pots, heavy books, and even your kids. While holding the object, squeeze tightly and curl your wrists upward, then reverse the position and extend your wrists backward.

# SHOW OFF YOUR GUNS

Your arms will get worked every time you pull, push, and grip anything. Whether hitting a hard bench press, carrying a child, or doing work around the house or yard, the arms are contributing to the strength required for those tasks. So why isolate them? For some, the thought of having chiseled arms just feels good. Certainly, the biceps and triceps can be separated, and you can work one over the other if you think you need that little extra, but training your entire arm means you will get that perfect shape, nice lines, and the strength you need to carry out your everyday tasks. If you hit them hard, your pistols will grow and ultimately become full-fledged guns. But even if that is not your goal, each of these mini workouts make a good training session to build that much-needed strength. Be careful, though; working your guns hard may result in a super pump, and it may take hours before your arms become usable again, but this is also a good time to show them off. These routines are designed to be quick, efficient, and straight to the point. Choose one routine, complete each set before moving to the next exercise, and your arms should get everything they need.

| Exercise | Number of sets | Reps per set | Rest between sets |
|---|---|---|---|
| **Routine 1** | | | |
| Supine triceps extension | 2 | 10 | 90 sec. |
| Dip | 2 | 10 | 90 sec. |
| 21s* | 2 | 7, 7, 7 | 90 sec. between full sets |
| Cable curl | 2 | 10 | 60 sec. |
| Wrist curl (palms down to work extensors) | 3 | 10 | 60 sec. |
| **Routine 2** | | | |
| Close-grip bench press | 2 | 12 | 90 sec. |
| Triceps push-down | 2 | 8 | 60 sec. |
| Straight bar curl | 2 | 12 | 90 sec. |
| Isolated dumbbell curl | 2 each arm | 8 | 60 sec. |
| Wrist curl (palms down to work extensors) | 3 | 12 | 60 sec. |
| **Routine 3** | | | |
| Overhead triceps extension | 2 each arm | 8 | 90 sec. |
| Cable reverse-grip triceps pull-down | 2 each arm | 12 | 60 sec. |
| Reverse-grip barbell curl | 2 | 8 | 90 sec. |
| Dumbbell curl | 2 | 12 | 60 sec. |

*For each set, perform 7 reps of half of the movement, 7 reps of the other half of the movement, and 7 reps of the complete movement one after another.

# 10

# CORE

Some trainers suggest that the core is its own independent part of the body. However, when you move, lift, pull, carry, throw, kick, punch, or hold anything, you push your feet toward the ground and transfer that force to your legs or arms via the connecting structures of your core. Thus, training the core is important, but it's not more important than strengthening the lower body. Additionally, the term *core* is often used to refer only to the abdominal region, but really your hips, abs, lower and upper back, and even pecs can act as part of your core. Since the pecs, lats, and hips are covered in other chapters, this chapter focuses on abdominal and lower back muscles.

The main role of the abdominal muscles is trunk flexion (allows you to sit up) and pelvic stabilization (allows you to dance without falling over). The main abdominal muscle that runs down the middle of your body is the rectus abdominis. The obliques on the sides of your body allow you to twist. The transverse abdominis runs across your abdominal region to provide support for posture and movement.

Soreness and injury in the lower back can have a profound effect on training, sport performance, and everyday life. Nearly 80 percent of all people will experience back problems at some point in their lifetime. Although most injuries are just strains, major problems can also occur. Many injuries can be prevented by strengthening the lower back muscles, so light back work should be incorporated into all programs.

Several myths exist about how to train the core. First, spot reduction—losing weight in one specific area of the body—is a fallacy. Second, you don't need expensive machines to work your abs or back. Third, you don't have to have a six-pack to have strong abs.

Most movements in daily life and sporting activity require the simultaneous contraction of both the abs and lower back. As a result, combined core exercises are becoming more popular. The "more to choose and use" section of this chapter presents a variety of these types of exercises on pages 124 through 135. Since the core musculature often contracts to stabilize the entire body, static hold exercises seem to do a good job at increasing core strength. But again, you should do a combination of both static and dynamic exercises to benefit both appearance and function.

## Crunch

For many years, this exercise was called a sit-up, but it has been modified to prevent neck and lower back injuries. Research shows that crunches, also known as curl-ups, activate all abdominal muscles as much as any other exercise. In fact, crunches cause greater activation of the abs than most ab machines advertised on TV.

1. Lie on your back with your knees bent and together or slightly apart, your feet flat on the ground about shoulder-width apart. You can perform this exercise with your hands by your sides. If you place your hands behind your head, do not pull on your neck when you curl up. The extra strain may damage the neck vertebrae.

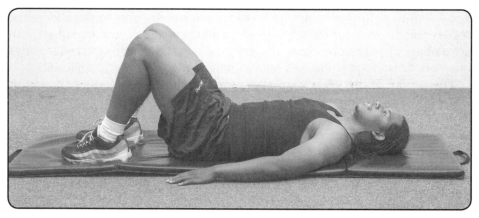

Starting position with hands at sides

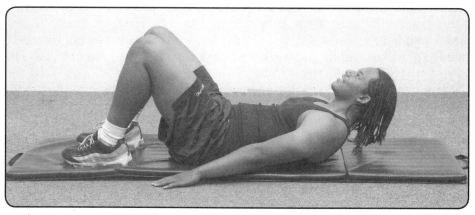

Curl up

2. Curl your trunk up to the point at which the middle of your back comes off the floor, but keep your lower back touching the floor. Perform the movement slowly. Jerky movements will bypass the abdominal muscles in favor of the much stronger hip flexors.

3. Squeeze at the top position for two counts, then slowly return to the starting position.

Once you have progressed to the point where you can perform many repetitions without losing proper form, you can increase the intensity of the crunch by extending your arms to your sides.

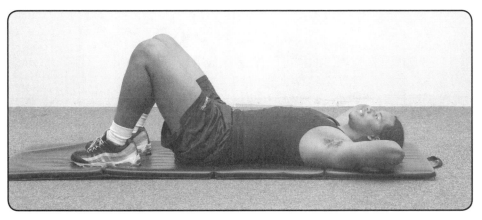

Starting position with hands behind head

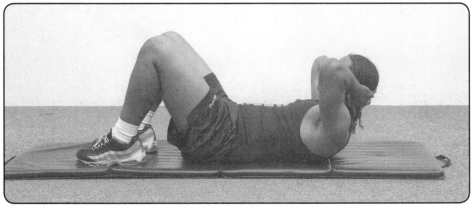

Curl up

# Back Extension

Back extensions, also called hyperextensions or hypers, work the lower back from a bent-over position. Straightening the body involves contracting the lower back muscles (as well as the glutes and even the hamstrings). Most gyms have a special bench for back extensions that places your body parallel to the ground. Another type of back extension bench positions your body at a 45 degree angle. For either bench, you can do the exercise with no resistance except body weight. To add more resistance, you can attach resistance tubing around your upper back or use a specially designed bench (if your gym has one) that allows you to adjust the resistance.

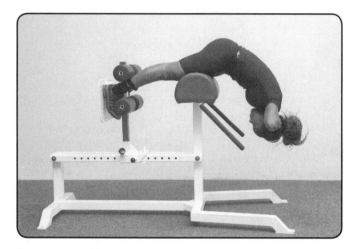

Starting position

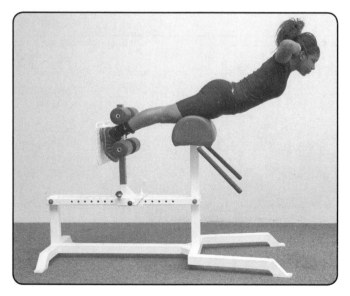

Extend upward

1. Position yourself on the bench so that the front of your legs are resting on the main pad of the bench with your hips just past the end of the bench and your feet fixed firmly in the supports. Lower your torso down so that the top of your head is pointing to the ground and so your legs and torso form about a 90 degree angle. Position your arms behind your head, beside you, across your chest, or extended out in front of you.
2. Squeeze your lower back muscles while extending upward until your body is straight.
3. Hold at the extended straight position for two counts. Slowly return to the starting position.

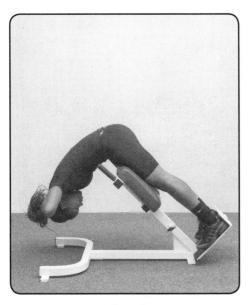

Starting position for alternative bench

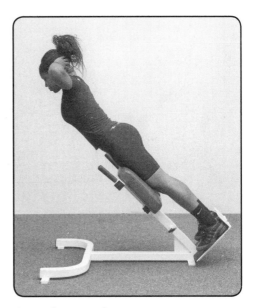

Extend upward

## Twisting Crunch

The most popular variation of a crunch is a twisting curl-up, which activates the obliques a little more. Slow, precise movement is the key. If you move too quickly, you won't work the abs.

1. Lie on your back, knees bent. Put your hands behind your head or over your ears and flare your elbows out to your sides.
2. Curl up, but twist at the waist as you near the top of the movement, moving one elbow toward the opposite knee.
3. Repeat on the other side.

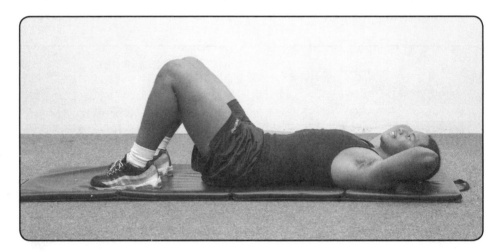

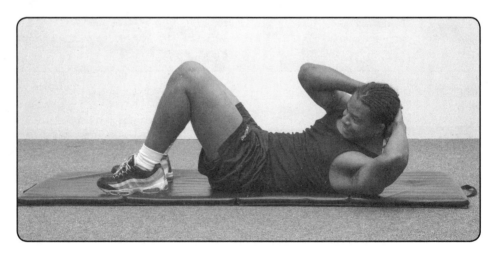

## Side Bend

The side bend also concentrates more on the obliques.

1. Stand with your feet shoulder-width apart, knees slightly bent.
2. With a dumbbell in each hand, arms straight at your sides, slowly lean side to side, accentuating the range of motion. Both sets of obliques will work in each direction as you lower and raise.

If you prefer, you can work one side at a time. Hold one dumbbell, and place the other hand behind your head for optimal balance.

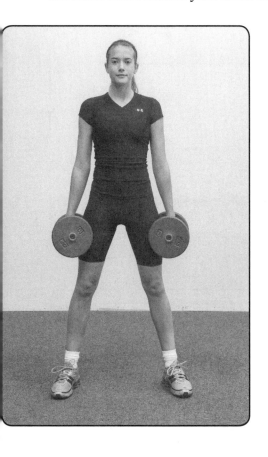 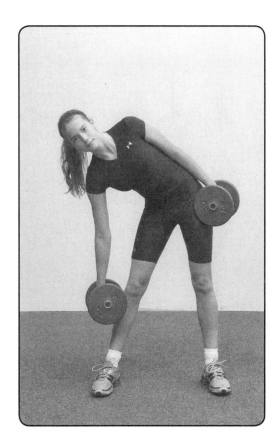

## Pelvic Raise

The pelvic raise is safe and effective at increasing the work on the lower abs while still working your entire abdominal region, although you should not perform this exercise if you have a sore back.

1. Lie on your back. Raise your legs, crossing your ankles and bending your knees slightly. The soles of your feet should point toward the ceiling.
2. Contract your abs, raising your buttocks off the ground.
3. Hold at the top of the movement for two counts. Don't expect a lot of movement; the actual amount may be only a few inches (several centimeters). Do not try to increase the movement by thrusting your hips into the air.

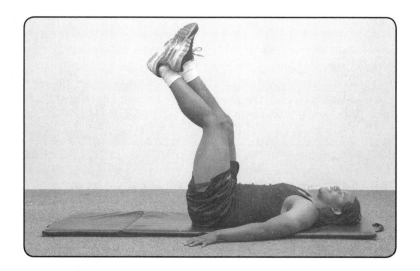

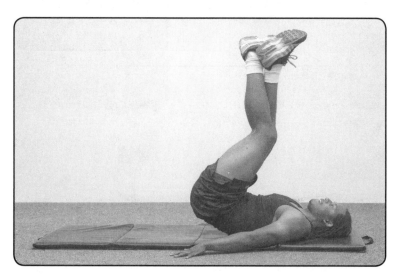

# Reverse Crunch

Although there is little proof that the lower abs can be truly isolated, it certainly feels that way when performing this crunch variation. Without a doubt it does tax the entire abdominal muscle wall, and provided that your lower back is injury free, it is a great way to target your abs.

1. Lie on your back with your head, shoulders, and butt against the ground. Raise your legs off the ground, crossing your ankles and bending your knees to 90 degrees.
2. Pull your knees toward your chest, pulling your buttocks off the ground by squeezing your abs.
3. Hold for two counts then return to the start.

Variations include the double ab crunch and the med ball crunch. The double ab crunch combines the actions of the curl-up crunch and the reverse crunch so that you are simultaneously pulling your chest and hips off the ground and bringing your knees to your elbows. Some people call this the clam crunch because the motion resembles a clam closing. The other variation is to trap a med ball or small stability ball between your hamstrings and calves. Then do your reverse crunch with the ball behind your knees during the movement.

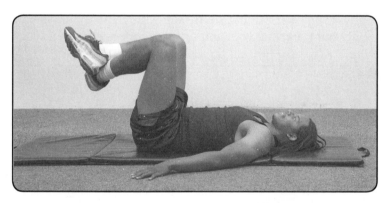

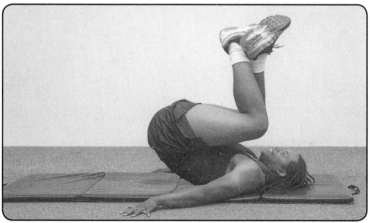

# Romanian Deadlift

A full deadlift is an exercise practiced by powerlifters for sheer strength. Coaches and trainers prefer to modify the deadlift by using a version known as the Romanian deadlift that takes a little pressure off the lower back. The Romanian deadlift requires good foundational strength and extremely good technique. The key is to keep the bar as close to your body as possible. If the bar travels too far away from your body or your form deteriorates, you may do considerable damage to your back. Do not do this exercise if your back is sore.

1. Stand with your feet about shoulder-width apart, perpendicular to the barbell, the bar resting on the floor across your shins. Bend at your waist, keeping about 10 to 20 degrees of knee flexion. Grasp the bar just wider than shoulder-width, with the palms turned toward you. Keep your arms fully extended during the entire movement. Stick your chest out, and pull up on the bar to reduce any slack in your legs or arms.

2. Slowly pull the bar up, keeping your arms locked and your back flat. Pull the bar along your legs until it is at waist height, with your arms fully extended. Keep the bar as close to your body as possible during the entire lift.

3. From the extended position, slowly lower the barbell; do not drop it. Proper control is essential. The torso should remain tight during the entire lift.

For a body-weight variation, use the same movement but without the barbell. Use only the weight of your upper torso for resistance.

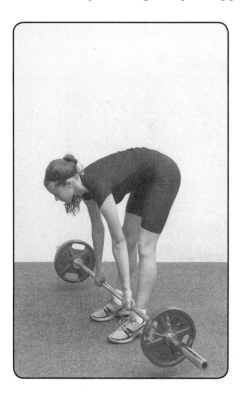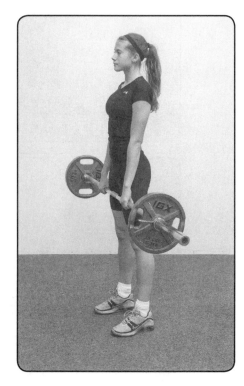

# Fire Hydrant and Rotational Fire Hydrant

The position of this exercise forces your abdominal and lower back muscles to engage to stabilize your hips. Although this is often considered a core exercise, you can also use it to work on your glutes and surrounding hip muscles.

1. Place your hands and knees on the floor so that your weight is evenly dispersed. Position your back so it is parallel to the floor and perfectly straight.
2. Raise the knee of your right leg out to your side. The movement is aptly named after the position a male dog takes when he is relieving himself. Hold your knee out to the side at 90 degrees for two counts before returning under control. Don't allow your torso to rotate at all during the movement.

A rotational fire hydrant refers to rotating the hip (not the torso). The exercise is performed the same way as the regular fire hydrant, except that you perform small circles with your hip when your knee is up and out to the side. Keep your knee at 90 degrees during the movement. Another option is to make larger circles with your knee at a 45-degree angle. Perform two or three circles, then bring your leg back down and repeat for 9 more reps (10 in total) before switching legs.

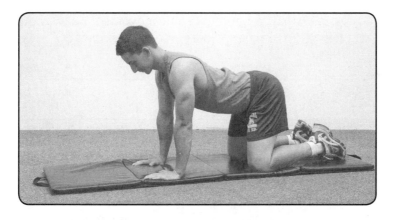

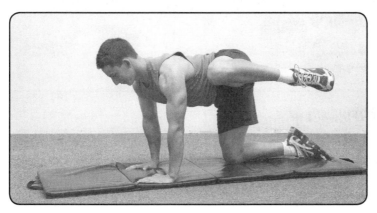

## Plank

The plank is a great total core exercise requiring co-contraction (simultaneous firing) of the stabilizing musculature to maintain proper balance. This is a static exercise that should be held for 30 seconds to a minute.

1. Start by lying facedown on the ground with your weight on your elbows and forearms. Be sure your elbows are directly under your shoulders and not tucked under your chest.

2. Lift your body off the ground, forming a bridge so that your weight is on your forearms and toes. Keep your torso as tight as possible. Don't raise your buttocks or let your torso sag; instead, make a completely straight line (a plank) with your body.

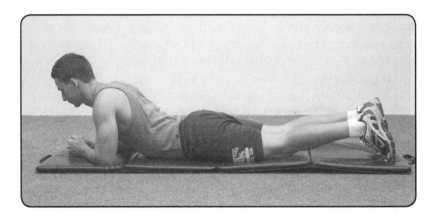

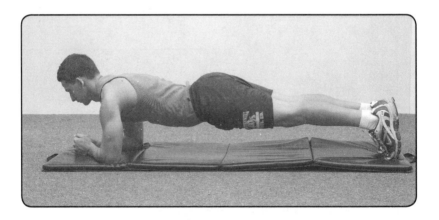

# Elbow to Hand Plank Lift

Since almost everything we do in life has a moving component, a great way to activate your core in a dynamic (moving) strengthening exercise is to take the regular plank and perform transfers (a fancy term for moving from one level to another). Perform 10 to 20 repetitions.

1. Start with your body in plank position (weight on your forearms and toes, with the torso in a straight line).
2. Keeping your torso perfectly tight, press up on one hand and then the other and extend your arms to move into push-up position.
3. Hold at the top for two counts, and then lower yourself back down to your elbows one hand at a time.
4. Repeat this sequence, keeping a good rhythm that increases speed but maintains a tight plank.

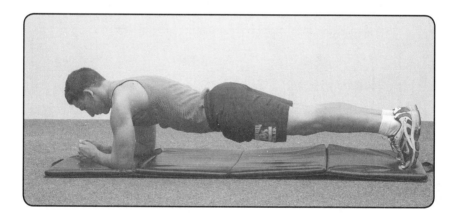

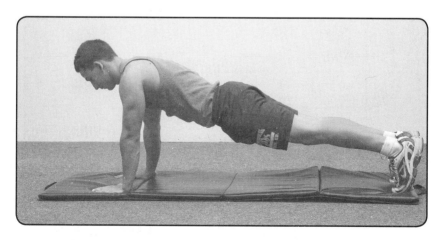

## Lateral Plank Raise

The lateral plank raise is definitely an advanced core exercise requiring considerable balance and strength. This exercise expands on the previous planks by introducing an unstable base on only one foot and one hand. You can do your reps to the same side or you can alternate, just make sure you don't wobble back and forth. A good target goal is 10 reps per side.

1. Start in a regular push-up position.
2. Rotate your weight to the right and roll onto your right foot. Simultaneously place your weight on the right hand, and raise your left arm out to the side.
3. In the finish position, your body forms the letter T, with your left arm fully extended and pointing to the ceiling; the entire front of your body is perpendicular to the ground.
4. Lower yourself back to the push-up position under control.

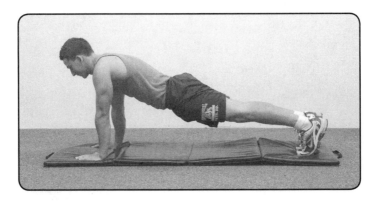

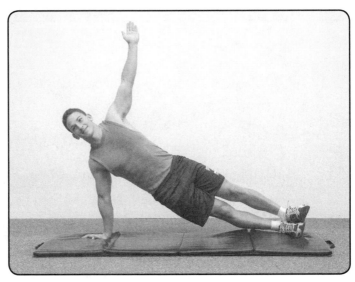

## Superman

Quickly becoming a common staple in many exercise programs, the aptly named superman focuses on total core activity. It starts with a dynamic contraction to get to the superman position and then requires strong static stabilization to maintain the hold.

1. Lie facedown on your belly with your arms extended past your head and legs fully stretched out.
2. While simultaneously contracting your glutes, hamstrings, and shoulders, lift your arms and legs off the ground. You should be balanced on your midsection and forming an exaggerated position that resembles Superman flying.
3. Hold for two counts, then return to the ground. When raising up, your entire torso should be tight, and both your knees and upper arms should come off the ground.

An alternative to the superman is the super T. The action is the same except that your arms are out to your sides rather than overhead.

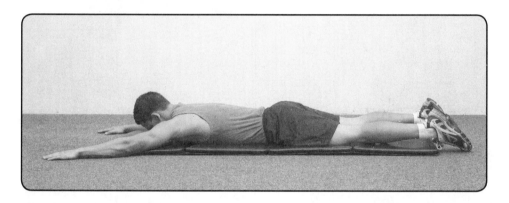

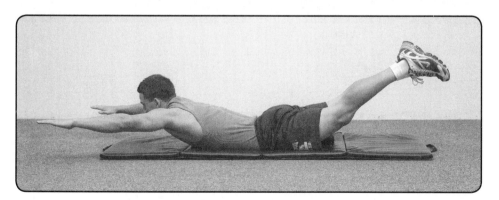

## Standing Rotational Twist

Since most daily activities involve standing, moving, and twisting, a great way to train the core, work on balance, and increase overall strength is to use resistance while performing a movement that incorporates the entire core.

1. Grab a med ball, a dumbbell, tubing, or a pulley cable system. Stand upright with your legs about twice as wide as shoulder width. Extend your arms directly out in front while grabbing the implement. Keep your arms locked and extended at shoulder height.

2. Rotate at the hips so that your entire upper body is facing sideways.

3. Twist back and forth to activate the entire torso.

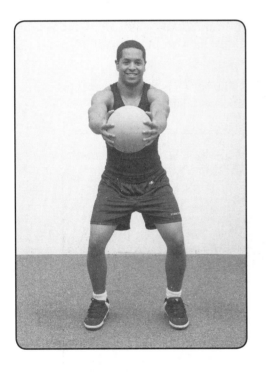 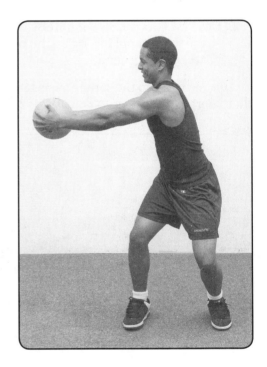

# Axe Chop

This is another great standing exercise that requires the entire body to participate. You can do this exercise with med balls, dumbbells, tubing, or a pulley cable system. Axe chops are a tough exercise and should be performed slowly at first until the move is perfected.

1. Stand upright with your legs about twice as wide as shoulder width. Extend your arms overhead while grabbing the med ball. Keep your arms locked and extended.

2. Rotate from shoulder to opposite knee, going across the body as if you are chopping wood. Keep your body tight, and bend over at the waist to perform this move.

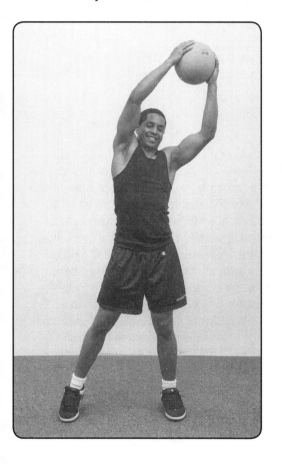
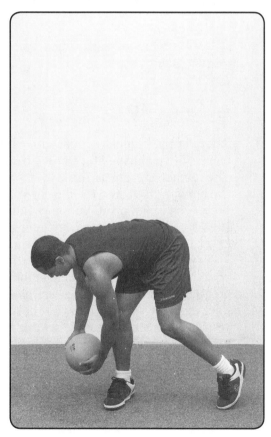

# TAKE IT TO THE GYM

## Slow Down to Tone the Abs

To train your abs better than ever, remember this one piece of advice: Slow down the movement. During crunches, imagine one end of a chain is attached to your rib cage, and someone at the other end is cranking you up one link at a time. Allow yourself to be slowly pulled up, completely contracting your abs one segment at a time. By slowing down the movement, you force the abs to work harder by removing the momentum generated by other muscles.

Keep your torso erect, and don't tuck your chin into your chest. To develop abdominal endurance, perform more reps. If strength is your goal, increase the resistance by altering your arm position or adding weight. Having a gym buddy press against you while you try to do crunches may be a good challenge. Advanced lifters can use medicine balls for an additional abdominal challenge.

Do not work the abs when your back is sore. Take your time, and be patient. Being able to see your six-pack may take much longer than its actual development.

## Don't Break Your Back

Safety is the biggest concern for all back exercises. Perform all back exercises slowly. During straight-leg deadlifts, keep the bar close to your body. The farther the bar is from your body, the more tension will be placed on the lumbar discs, and the harder you will have to work to control the weight. When you finish a set, you may want to stretch your lower back and take a slightly longer rest period. For a quick stretch, grab hold of a machine or post, extend your arms, and round your upper back by leaning away from the pole.

As with all exercises, proper technique is a must. Contract the abs to keep your torso erect; this will help stabilize your entire body. Do not use a weight belt when performing back exercises unless a physician tells you to do so. Back exercises strengthen your core; the belt will reduce this effect. Respect your lower back; do not work your back if it is sore. If the soreness persists for more than two days, see a physician.

# TRAIN AT HOME

## Core Training Creativity

There is no excuse for flabby abs! Since most ab and back exercises use just your body weight, you can do your core exercises virtually anywhere. Your home can become the perfect gym, but creating additional resistance requires a little imagination. Instead of dumbbells, use soup cans or other heavier objects. In fact, give yourself a challenge by selecting an expensive vase and trying to keep it from falling. If it does, however, I take absolutely no responsibility for damages! Using towels, tubing, and other forms of resistance along with a couch or bed, you can do every exercise in this chapter in your home. For those wanting a real challenge, try a plank with a young child on your back. Get imaginative, but try to focus on those all-important core muscles, and your flabs will turn to abs in no time.

# DO MORE FOR YOUR CORE

You can add core routines to the end of your workout, do them alone, or intersperse core exercises throughout your workout. These mini workouts are designed to strengthen your body for both static movements, postural activity, and functional daily dynamic movements. Routine 1 is a floor-based routine that can be done anywhere, anytime, such as right before bed. Routines 2 and 3 combine several elements that may be added to your leg or back training days.

| Exercise | Number of sets | Reps per set | Rest between sets |
|---|---|---|---|
| **Routine 1** | | | |
| Crunch | 2 | 12 | 60 sec. |
| Reverse crunch | 2 | 12 | 60 sec. |
| Twisting crunch | 2 | 12 | 60 sec. |
| Superman | 2 | 12 | 90 sec. |
| **Routine 2** | | | |
| Plank | 2 | 1 30-sec. hold per set | 90 sec. between holds |
| Lateral plank raise | 3 each side | 8 | 60 sec. |
| Rotational fire hydrant | 3 each side | 10 | 60 sec. |
| **Routine 3** | | | |
| Romanian deadlift | 2 | 12 | 90 sec. |
| Back extension | 2 | 10 | 90 sec. |
| Axe chop | 2 | 10 | 75-90 sec. |
| Standing rotational twist | 2 each side | 10 | 75-90 sec. |

# 11

# GLUTES AND HIPS

Everyone wants to have a tighter backside. The gluteus maximus, gluteus medius, and gluteus minimus, collectively referred to as the glutes, make up the major muscles of the buttocks. These muscles along with the hamstrings help pull the leg back. The gluteus medius, with the help of a few other muscles such as the tensor fasciae latae and the sartorius on the outer thigh, moves the leg to the side. Several other muscles, including the gracilis and adductor magnus of the inner thigh, bring the leg back in. The psoas major and iliacus muscles at the front of the hip help bring the knee to the chest. The entire group of muscles acts on the hip for both movement and stabilization.

Infomercials promoting home machines have led many to believe that glute, hip, and leg muscles can be individually targeted to burn off excess fat. Furthermore, some machines tout that they can isolate the glutes, making them firmer and tighter. Sorry to burst that bubble, but spot reduction is a fallacy. And as far as tighter glutes, even most health club butt-blaster machines work the quadriceps muscles of the leg first rather than the hip muscles. Only isolated hip extension, adduction, and abduction can truly target the glutes. Since the gluteus maximus is responsible for hip extension, one major movement can hit the glutes hard and work all of the surrounding musculature.

## Leg Press

Before the creation of the leg press, the squat—heralded as the king of all exercises—was a mainstay for all strength- and mass-building programs. However, since the squat is not easy to learn, we'll begin with the leg press. The squat is covered in chapter 12 with the quadriceps exercises, but it requires significant contribution from the glutes. There are several different kinds of leg presses, but all will work the muscles adequately. The key is to select a machine that is comfortable and takes pressure off your back. Leg presses work just about every muscle in the lower body, although the glutes and adductors will work the most.

Depending on the machine, the movement may begin with your knees at your chest or your legs fully extended. In either case, when the legs are flexed, the thighs should be parallel with the footpads. During the extension phase, you can gently lock your knees; do not snap your knees into place.

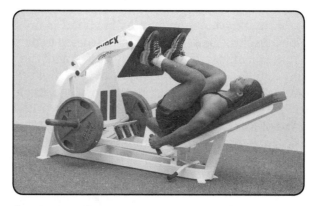

Starting position

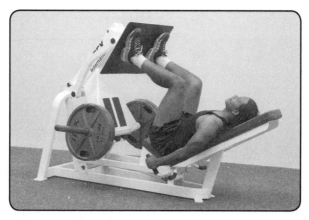

Slowly extend legs

1. For a machine that starts with the legs flexed, begin with your feet higher up on the footpads, toes pointing out slightly. Foot position is vital for proper alignment during the lift and for emphasizing specific muscles. Pointing the toes out helps the body follow its normal path and prevents the knees from bending and pinching in. The farther apart your legs are, the more the adductors will have to work during the movement.

2. Slowly and steadily extend your legs. Do not bounce at the top. Do not let your knees track past your toes. The lower legs should be perpendicular to the footpad. Contract your abs and lower back to keep your body stable. Maintain an erect posture. Do not let your lower back round, and keep your head up and chest out.

3. Pause for two counts at the top of the movement to keep momentum from rushing the flexion stage. Slowly bend your knees, bringing them close to your chest. The flexion stage may be slightly faster than the extension, but it should still be under control.

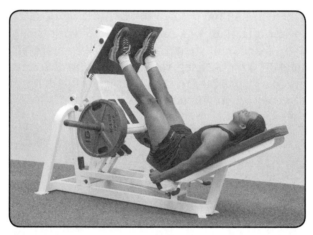

Pause at fully extended position

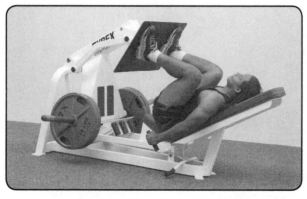

Return to starting position

## Step-Up

Balance, coordination, and athleticism sum up the requirements for this important exercise. Since most people need to negotiate stairs on a daily basis, at first this exercise seems pretty straightforward, and it may be hard to see how it can benefit. When done correctly, this movement will get help from the quads but can be a punisher for your hips. Taking a normal step or adding steps to an aerobics class does not do a great job of firming and strengthening the hips, unlike a true strength step-up. Aim for standard bench or box heights, which fall between 12 and 18 inches (30 and 45 cm). You can use a bench or any device if you can get a firm base of support for at least one leg.

1. Start with one leg up on top of the box so the thigh is parallel with the ground. Lean forward slightly while pushing downward on the leg on the box. Do not push off of your back foot.

2. Raise your entire body up until your leg is fully extended. Your trail leg should drag along the box at first for stability, but as you get comfortable, you will want to keep it out of the way to really emphasize the action of the glutes on the lead leg.

3. Slowly lower yourself back down to the starting position. At this point you can either alternate legs or continue to work the same leg until a complete set is accomplished. If you choose to work one leg at a time, don't bounce off your back leg; rather, take control and force the lead leg to do as much as possible. To create a bigger challenge, use dumbbells or even a barbell when you do this move.

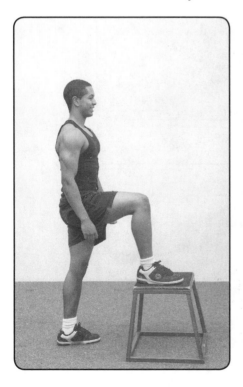 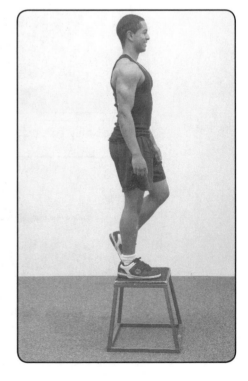

## Hip Extension

Most hip extensor machines can be adjusted for a larger range of motion. The larger the range of motion, the more the glutes are involved. Set the roll pad as far up as possible so that your knees are close to your chest. Machines that require you to lie down generally work both legs at the same time. Machines that require you to stand work one leg at a time. Whether standing or lying, as long as the hip has a long range of extension, your glutes will get the necessary work.

1. Lie on the bench with the roller pad under your knees. Move your body under the pad so that your knees are at your chest.

2. Press down on the pad, extending your hips and legs completely. Keep the torso erect during the movement, and do not thrust the legs back violently.

3. Pause for two counts at your point of full hip extension (your body fully extended) before returning the legs to the starting position.

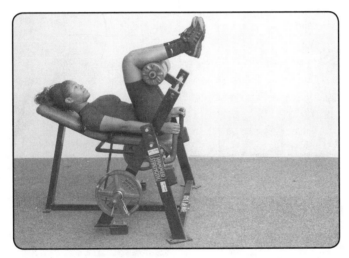

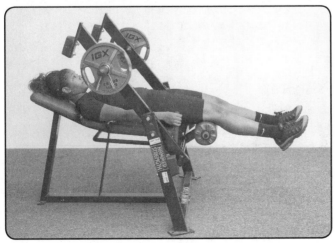

## Low-Cable Kickback

A low pulley attached to a multistation cable machine can be used for a variety of exercises to work the glutes and hips. The low-cable kickback and three other low-pulley exercises (side-cable lift, adductor cable lift, and hip flexor cable lift) are referred to as the four-way hip. For the low-cable kickback, add a low pulley strap to a multistation cable machine so that the pulley is on the floor. A simple belt will do if no special strap is available.

1. Stand facing the weight stack. Hook the pulley around the ankle of your working leg. Use the other leg for support.

2. Pull the strapped leg back against the resistance. Maintain proper posture throughout the lift. The greater the range of motion, the more the glutes will be worked.

3. Return to the starting position by slowly bringing your leg forward.

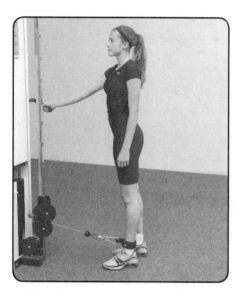 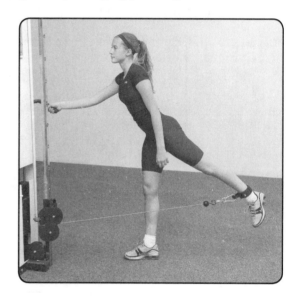

# Side-Cable Lift

You can also use the low pulley to target the outer thigh, working the adductors, abductors, and hip flexors.

1. Stand next to the weight stack, and hook the pulley around the ankle of your outside leg.
2. Pull your leg to the side, away from your body.
3. Slowly return to the starting position, resisting the weight as you lower your leg.

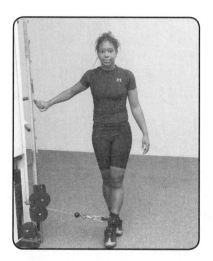 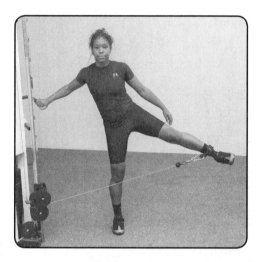

## Adductor Cable Lift

The low pulley can also be used to work the adductors of the inner thigh.

1. Stand beside the weight stack. Hook the pulley around the ankle of your inner leg.
2. Pull your leg across your body, away from the weight stack.
3. Slowly return to the starting position, resisting the pull of the weight.

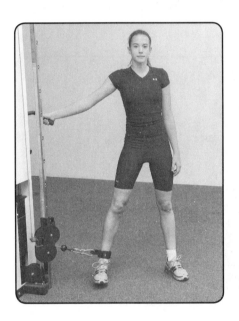 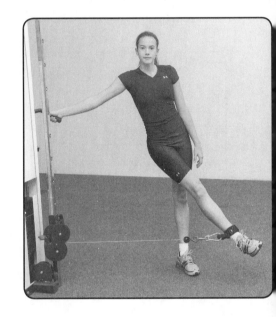

# Hip Flexor Cable Lift

Most people do not consider working the hip flexors since they are not as visible as the buns, and they do not hold extra fat. But they are important for everyday function and should not be overlooked. For stability, position a bench on your nonworking side and rest your hand on it.

1. With the low pulley on the cable machine, turn away from the weight stack. Hook the low pulley around the ankle of your working leg.
2. Kick your working leg straight out in front, working the hip flexors.
3. Slowly return to the starting position.

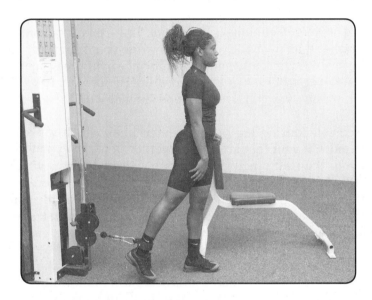

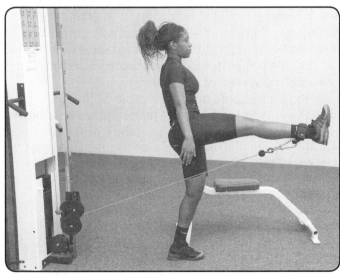

# TAKE IT TO THE GYM

## Help Your Hips

Strengthening the entire hip capsule will improve all aspects of balance and strength. Toning these muscles will not only give your hips and backside a nice shape but also help increase speed and strength for lower body activities. Having strong muscles around the hip also decreases the potential for hip fractures later in life. The key to tight buns is to work deep into the muscle and increase the range of motion. If leg presses are too hard on your knees, try the isolated single-leg movements. Don't jerk the weight; use smooth, regular contractions. Work the hip in all four directions instead of focusing on having a tight backside or thigh.

During leg presses, technique is important. Try to push yourself away from the weight rather than push the weight away from you. Your focus shifts from fear of being crushed by the weight to dominance over the weight. Additionally, make sure the machine is adjusted properly for you. If it doesn't feel right, then it probably isn't. Have someone familiar with the machine adjust it for you.

Foot placement during leg presses determines which muscles will be worked the most. If your feet are close together, generally you will work the outside of your thighs more. If your feet are wide apart, you will emphasize the inner thighs, hamstrings, and glutes. Although the difference may be small, changing your foot position will help improve overall hip stability and add variety. If you are primarily using the leg press or even a squat for hip strength and shape, then take the wide stance every time.

In most cases, the movement in weight training should be at a regular, smooth, and even pace for ultimate muscle strength and shape. However, athletes can use a more explosive approach, forcing the hips to respond more rapidly and increasing overall power in strides and jumps. Once your technique is well perfected, pick up your rep pace, gradually at first, until you are capable of performing your reps with maximal speed. You don't have to always perform explosive reps, nor should you; however, incorporating a few faster moves into your program will help improve your overall stride and put a jump in your step when you hit those stairs.

You will have to endure some pretty tough workouts to see good definition in the glutes and legs. Trembling legs are just a minor symptom of hard work. Make it through these initially difficult workouts, and your training volume will improve—and so will your results. However, be smart and listen to your body. If your back is sore, discontinue these exercises. Patience is a virtue. You didn't get out of shape in a day, and you won't get back into shape in a day. Think of this area as a long-term project.

# TRAIN AT HOME

## Target Your Tush

As we have seen before, modifying your regular exercises by using resistance bands is a great choice for home-based programs. Using a band for your four-way hip work (inner, outer, front, back) might be easy in your house, but exercises such as leg presses may be much more difficult. Your body weight is enough to give you a real challenge, though, so body-weight exercises are the rule for the hips and quads when working at home.

In the case of trying to isolate your tush, it may be hard to find an exercise that does not incorporate your legs, but that's okay. When working at home, just alternating foot position in general exercises may do the trick. For many, using weight and performing deep knee squats that are lower than parallel will be quite a challenge, but it is easier when using body weight. Taking a wide stance forces the adductors to get more involved, but when you hit parallel or below, your quads rely on your glutes to get you up—you can't extend your hips without them (the glutes). So the number one exercise for home-based training is wide-stance deep squats because they work both your butt and quads, but more important, they provide a serious challenge for even the strongest of individuals.

Using proper upper body squat position (see chapter 12 for more information), start with your legs twice as wide as shoulder width or even wider. As you descend, push your butt backward until your body reaches parallel or just below. At the bottom, drive hard into the ground, bringing your hips in on the way up until you are fully extended. Pause for two counts, and then hit 11 more grueling reps. If you can't go deep, work on it, but at the very least try for a few reps and really feel your tush scream.

# COMBO LEG ROUTINES

For a complete hip and lower body workout, simply do a few sets of leg presses plus the four-way hip exercises (low-cable kickbacks, side-cable lifts, adductor cable lifts, and hip flexor cable lifts). However, several other combinations include the quadriceps and hamstrings. The table shows several good routines. Routine 1 is a good general program for overall lower body development. Routine 2 works a few extra muscles and may be a good way to work everything if you are short on time.

| Exercise | Number of sets | Reps per set | Rest between sets |
|---|---|---|---|
| **Routine 1** | | | |
| Leg press | 2 | 8 | 2 min. |
| Step-up | 2 each leg | 12 | 90 sec. |
| Hip extension | 2 each leg | 10 | 60 sec. |
| Hip flexor cable lift | 2 each leg | 10 | 60 sec. |
| **Routine 2** | | | |
| Step-up | 2 each leg | 8 | 2 min. |
| Leg press | 2 | 12 | 2 min. |
| Adductor cable lift | 2 each leg | 12 | 60 sec. |
| Side-cable lift | 2 each leg | 12 | 60 sec. |
| **Routine 3** | | | |
| Hip extension | 2 each leg | 10 | 90 sec. |
| Side-cable lift | 2 each leg | 10 | 90 sec. |
| Adductor cable lift | 2 each leg | 10 | 90 sec. |
| Hip flexor cable lift | 2 each leg | 10 | 90 sec. |

# 12

---

# QUADS

---

Muscle balance doesn't refer only to balance front to back. It also refers to balance top to bottom. Some lifters focus so much on upper body development that they neglect their chopstick-like legs. The quadriceps (or quads) in the upper legs are made up of four muscles. The vastus lateralis, vastus medialis, and vastus intermedius all help extend the lower leg at the knee. The rectus femoris crosses two joints: the hip, where it helps in hip flexion, and the knee, where it helps extend the lower leg. Although the quad muscles don't originate at the same point, they all come together at the kneecap.

There is much speculation about whether or not each individual quadriceps muscle can be isolated or stressed to a greater extent. Any evidence supporting the idea that you can develop your outer or inner quad muscles separately is mostly anecdotal at this point. However, solid research has shown that you can emphasize one quadriceps muscle over the others. The general method thought to target one of the quadriceps muscle heads more than another is to adjust the position of your feet. If time is of the essence, focus on the lifts themselves rather than manipulating your foot position. But if you have a little time, give it a try. Turning your foot outward may in fact engage your vastus medialis (inner quadriceps) more, while turning your foot inward may enhance vastus lateralis (outer quadriceps) activation. But remember, executing the lift correctly is always more important than trying to isolate a particular head.

## Squat

The squat, the king of all lifts, works the quads hard. Before attempting squats, you need proper base strength. Those with poor strength or flexibility should practice squats without weights before progressing to light weights. Beginners can learn the correct technique by using no weights and squatting down to a chair or box. For experienced lifters, after proper progression and regular training, squats can produce fabulous results.

Setting up and spotting may be the most important factor in making this lift work for you. You should always squat in a rack with safety stops to catch the weight if you fail, and you should have a spotter who can properly assist you. In general, spotting for lighter than maximal loads is best done by having the spotter apply a small force to the bar itself rather than interfere with the lifter. For heavier loads, your partner should stand directly behind you, giving you just enough room to descend properly, and should be braced to help with the lift by providing support around your waist and chest. If a big spot is needed, your partner will need to press his body up against yours and cross his arms across your chest to help you stand back up. Spotting this lift takes practice, and because of the close physical proximity of the lifter and spotter, you may prefer to have someone you know help you.

When lifting very heavy loads (which should be performed only by advanced lifters), you may need to have more than one spotter. If the weight is too heavy for you to lift even with a spotter, do not attempt the lift with the idea of bailing and using the safety stops to catch the weight.

1. To ensure safety, you should always enter the rack moving forward (from the opposite side where the weight is racked), take the weight off the rack, back up, do your set, and then walk back forward to rack the weights. When removing the weight from the rack, position the barbell across your traps and shoulders using a thumb-lock grip. Once you are set with the bar, stand up and take two small shuffle steps backward to clear the rack. Keep your head up, chin pointing forward, and chest out throughout the entire exercise. Your lower back will be slightly arched. Place your feet wider than shoulder-width apart, with your toes pointing out slightly.

2. Inhale deeply, and contract your abs and back muscles to stabilize your body. Begin to lower your body by thrusting your hips back. (A common mistake is to begin the movement by bending your knees, which can easily pull you out of position.)

3. Continue to lower your body by moving your hips back and bending at your knees and waist. Lower yourself until your thighs are nearly parallel to the floor. Keep your body tight and upright, and don't let your knees track past your toes. During the squat movement, your back should be flat, your chest and chin should be up, and you should be looking forward, not down. Do not let your back round at any time during the lift.

4. Pause for two counts at the bottom of the movement. To return to the starting position, exhale and powerfully thrust your hips under your body. Finish the rep by locking your knees, as long as you control it. Do not pop into a lockout.

From time to time it is a good idea to change your base of support when performing squats. By moving your feet out, you get a little more glute and adductor muscle (groin) activity, resulting in greater interior hip support. By moving your feet in closer, you get more outer quad (vastus lateralis) and abductor work, which strengthens the entire hip and knee. The execution of these advanced positions is identical to the standard squat, but you may have to adjust your range of motion to match your new body position. Also, these foot positions should be used only when sufficient back strength has been developed because they tend to increase the stress on the lower back. Perform your normal set of squats for two or three sets, then perform one additional set of each foot variation for complete glute and quad development.

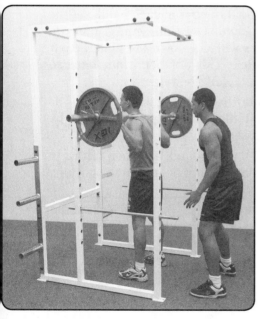

Starting position

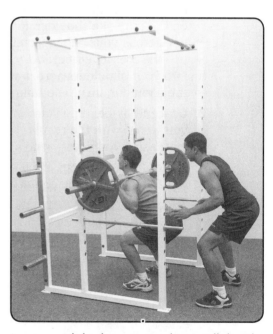

Lower until thighs are nearly parallel with floor

## Front Squat

At first glance, this exercise appears to simply move the bar from the back to the clavicle, but this little modification changes everything. When the bar is on your back, you can lean forward at the waist to counterbalance. This forward lean engages the hips, but seasoned lifters know that to isolate the quads, they need to remove the hips from the lift as much as possible. Because of bar position on the front squat, you are forced to take a more upright position (otherwise the bar would fall off or pull you forward), reducing hip demand and increasing quad load. Beginners will want to learn this exercise on a Smith machine or similar system before moving on to free weights. For this exercise, the bar should be adjusted on the rack at a height just lower than your clavicle so that you can step under it and stand up with enough room to clear the rack itself. As with regular squats, you can adjust your foot positions to emphasize different muscles.

1. Position yourself so that the bar is across your clavicle. Try to take a slightly wider than shoulder-width grip with your hands. People with greater arm mass or less flexibility may need to use the crossover method in which the arms cross over the top of the barbell so that each hand is on the opposite shoulder. If you can hold the bar in each hand, set the bar across your palms facing upward, and then close your grip. If you use the crossover method, your palms will face down and hold the bar into your shoulders across your clavicle. This position is not ideal, so the shoulder must help hold the bar.

2. Descend by bending your knees rather than starting with your hips as you would with the regular squat. Maintain a more upright position by increasing your knee-bend angle and keeping your torso tight.

3. Lower until your legs are parallel with the ground, and then return to the starting position. Again, as for all lifts, do not bounce at the bottom.

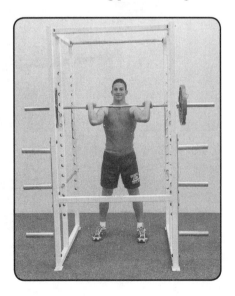 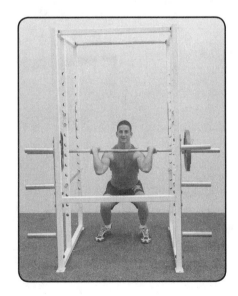

# Single-Leg Squat

Talk about a serious quad burn! This is one tough exercise that should be attempted only after you have mastered the technique of a regular squat. Although the movement for this exercise is similar to the squat, since the legs are isolated, it is harder to get hip activity because the glutes prefer to work in pairs when it comes to standing up from a deep position. You want to take a more upright position to further reduce hip demand and increase quad load. This exercise is primarily a body-weight movement, but adding dumbbells, barbells, or other forms of resistance is encouraged. Before adding resistance, as with any exercise, make sure your technique is perfect. Do 15 reps on one side and then switch to the other side. Listen to your quads beg for mercy.

1. Position yourself so that one leg can rest on a bench behind you. Your other leg has all your weight and is out in front as if you are doing a lunge.

2. Descend by bending your knee rather than starting with your hip, and maintain as upright a position as possible.

3. Keep your torso tight at all times, and go as deep as possible before pausing for two counts and returning to your starting position.

Those who have both great balance and strength can try to do this movement without supporting the nonworking leg. If you go without support, you can opt for the nonworking leg behind, giving you a slightly forward lean and less range of motion, but the true test is placing your nonworking leg straight out in front and going as deep as possible.

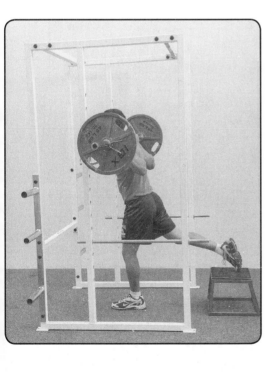 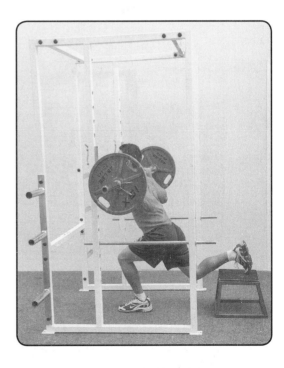

## Dumbbell Squat

Arguably, this exercise could go with hips or legs. Much of the emphasis will depend on where the dumbbells are hanging and how your torso is positioned (hip angle). If you take a narrow stance and hold the dumbbells close to your body, staying as upright as possible, your quads will let you know that they are the primary muscles working. Take a wider stance and get the dumbbells out in front a little (almost like the deadlift position), and Mr. Glutes will take charge. As for any squat, body control is the most important consideration.

1. Grab a pair of dumbbells and hang them beside you to emphasize your quads more. Grab a single dumbbell and hang it between your legs, taking a wide stance for a hip-dominant squat.

2. Descend under control to as deep as comfortable.

3. Pause for two counts, and return to the start.

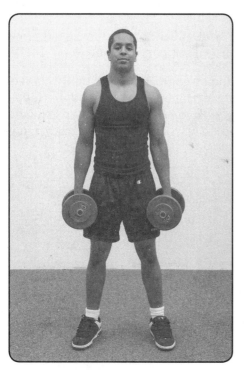 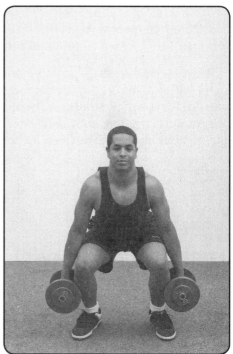

# Leg Extension

A leg workout is not complete without a few hard-fought reps on the leg extension machine. A leg extension machine can work each leg individually or both legs together, although it seems to be more challenging and beneficial to work both legs together.

1. Adjust the machine's seat so your knees are lined up directly with the machine arm's axis of rotation and your shins rest against the pad (legs start at about 90 degrees). Note your settings so you can use them later. If the machine has a belt, use it; you will need it when you work hard.

2. Push against the pad until your legs are fully extended and parallel to the ground. Either gently lock your knees or do not lock them at all. Keep the tension on your thighs the entire time. Do not throw the weight up; your body should remain in the machine.

3. After a brief pause, lower the weight back down slowly under control. Don't let the weight drop because this will decrease the work done by your quads.

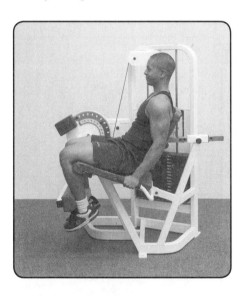 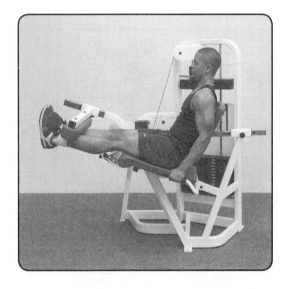

# Lunge

If you don't have access to a leg extension machine, lunges are a good choice. This lower body exercise has become popular with those looking to tone, tighten, and shape their legs. Lunges are often done by athletes and weekend warriors looking to gain balance and strength. Stationary lunges will tone the legs as well as train stability and balance. This exercise may look easy, but don't let it fool you.

1. Stand upright with your arms at your sides, one dumbbell in each hand. (Instead of dumbbells, you can use a barbell. Place the barbell across your traps and shoulders, using a thumb-lock grip.) Step forward with one foot a comfortable distance (about three feet or one meter). Keep your legs shoulder-width apart to help you balance the weight.

2. Bend the forward knee until the thigh is parallel to the floor and the rear knee just skims the ground. The lead knee should not track over the toes.

3. Pause for two counts at the bottom. Push back on the lead foot to return to the starting position.

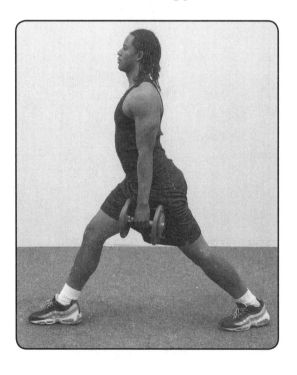
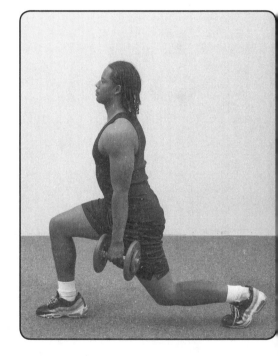

# Walking Lunge

Walking lunges are an advanced version of the stationary lunge. Do not perform walking lunges until you have mastered stationary lunges. The walking lunge has the same starting position as the stationary lunge.

1. Stand upright, arms at your sides, a dumbbell in each hand or a barbell across your shoulders. Step forward a comfortable distance (about three feet or one meter), keeping your legs shoulder-width apart.
2. Bend the forward knee until the thigh is parallel to the floor and the rear knee just skims the ground. The lead knee should not track over the toes.
3. Pause for two counts at the bottom. Lean slightly forward to generate forward momentum for the next rep.
4. Take a step forward with the back leg a comfortable distance, and bend the knee until the thigh is parallel to the floor. Continue for several steps.

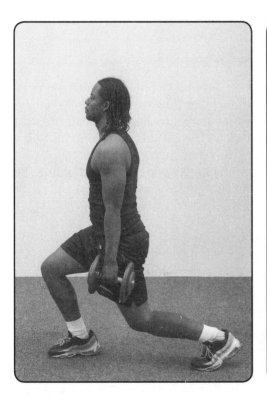
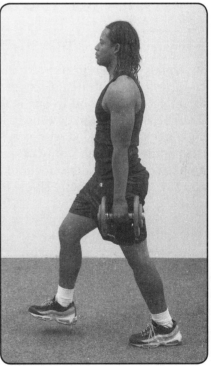

# TAKE IT TO THE GYM

## Tips for Quad Training

Two main tips can help you build your quads safely and effectively. First, do not use a belt, wrap, or special device to help you lift. Using a belt cheats the abdominal and lower back muscles out of their responsibility to protect and serve. Second, when you use a barbell, make sure the bar travels vertically up and down with little or no horizontal movement (except for walking lunges). Horizontal movement in either direction indicates flaws in technique.

When you are starting out, don't be afraid to use just your body weight to learn correct technique before moving on to weights. Don't feel that you have to lift huge weights to reap the benefits of weight training. More important than using heavy weights is controlling the weight and using proper technique. Make sure you have established good balance and technique before lifting with heavy weights.

# TRAIN AT HOME

## Attack Your Quads in Your Quarters

Several of the exercises shown in this chapter make good home-based exercises. Body-weight squats, lunges, and single-leg movements are all you need to get your body, and in particular your quads, in shape. Instead of using dumbbells, you could do these exercises with your kids on your back, wearing a backpack loaded with soup cans or other heavy items, or by placing the middle of a length of resistance tubing under your feet and holding the handles out to the sides at shoulder height. Find the method that works for you to help you perfectly shape those thighs.

# TONE THE THIGHS

The table shows a few good programs that work the quads. Remember, work hard, play later.

| Exercise | Number of sets | Reps per set | Rest between sets |
|----------|----------------|--------------|-------------------|
| **Routine 1** | | | |
| Squat | 2 | 8 | 2 min. |
| Single-leg extension | 2 each leg | 12 | 90 sec. between same leg |
| Leg press (see chapter 11) | 2 | 20 | 90 sec. |
| **Routine 2** | | | |
| Front squat | 2 | 8 | 2 min. |
| Walking lunge | 2 | 8 each leg | 2 min. |
| Leg extension | 2 | 12 | 90 sec. |
| **Routine 3** | | | |
| Single-leg squat | 2 each leg | 10 | 2 min. between same leg |
| Dumbbell squat | 2 | 12 | 90 sec. |
| Lunge | 2 each leg | 8 | 90 sec. |

# 13

# HAMSTRINGS

The hamstrings, the muscles that run up the back of the thigh, are crucial for support. They are the knee flexors, so they function opposite to the quadriceps. The three hamstring muscles cross both the hip and knee joints, making them responsible for both flexing the knee and pulling the leg back at the hip. These muscles act heavily in hip extension (see chapter 11) when the quads are not in optimal position. So although they compete against one another at the knee, if the knee is not needed, then the hamstrings will fire to help the glutes extend the hip.

The hamstrings, often referred to as the hammys or hams, are often neglected and undertrained and, as a result, are the most commonly strained muscle in the body. Proper development of the hamstrings will balance the body and reduce strain on the lower back. Lower back problems are often associated with weak and inflexible hamstrings. At first, when working the hamstrings, your lower back will likely get sore because those muscles will get a little extra work in some exercises. In time, the lower back will get stronger, and the hamstrings will make even greater gains.

# Lying Leg Curl

The most popular exercise for the hamstrings is definitely the lying leg curl. If possible, use a machine that allows for a slight bend in the hips. This decreases the likelihood of cheating and improves the isolation of the hamstrings. You can work each leg individually, but as with leg extensions, this exercise is more beneficial if you work both legs at the same time.

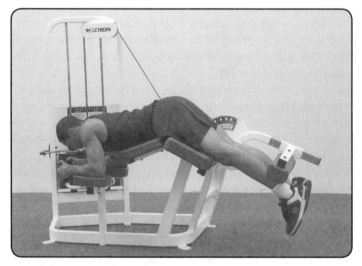

Staring position

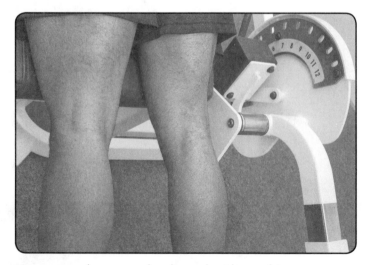

Knees must be properly aligned with machine

1. Lie facedown with your legs fully extended in the machine. The pad should rest just beneath your calf muscles. The position of your knees with respect to the machine arm's axis of rotation is extremely important. Line up your knees with the middle of the cam's axis of rotation. This ensures proper distribution of resistance from the machine.

2. With constant, even force, lift your heels to your buttocks, and squeeze your hamstrings and glutes at the top position. Hold for two counts, then release.

3. Lower the weight back to the starting position under control.

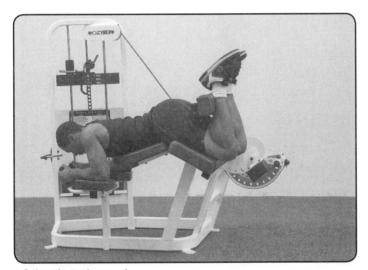

Lift heels to buttocks

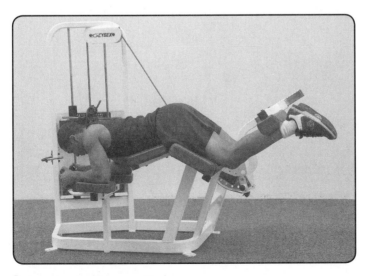

Return to starting position

## Seated Leg Curl

Many people prefer working the hammys in a seated position for comfort. From a strength standpoint, you are stronger seated than lying because of a slightly shorter range of motion. This is a great alternative to the lying leg curl and is much easier to get in and out of or to use advanced techniques, such as drop sets or slow training.

1. Begin with your legs straight out in front. The pad should rest against the Achilles tendons beneath your calf muscles.
2. Pull your legs back toward your buttocks as far as you can and hold.
3. Return to the starting position under control.

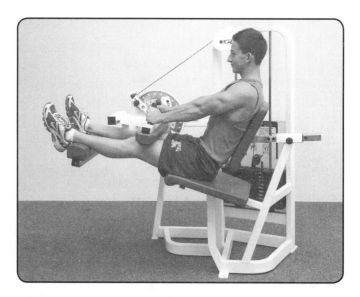

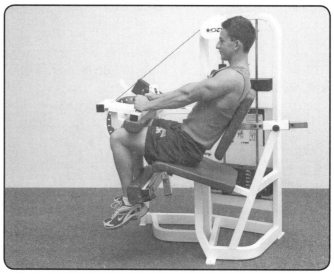

## Single-Leg Curl

If you like a challenge, try a standing single-leg curl. This exercise comple-ments the four-way hip described in chapter 11. Add a low pulley strap to a multistation cable machine so that the pulley is on the floor. (Another option is to do the lying leg curl with one leg at a time. Many gyms even have a single-leg curl machine.)

1. Stand facing the weight stack. Hook the pulley around the ankle of your working leg. Use the other leg for support.
2. Bend the knee of the working leg, bringing your heel toward your but-tocks. Maintain proper posture and balance. If necessary, hold onto something stable to keep your balance.
3. Pause for two counts at the end of the movement before returning to the starting position under control.

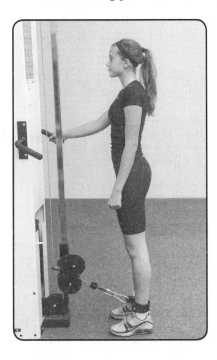
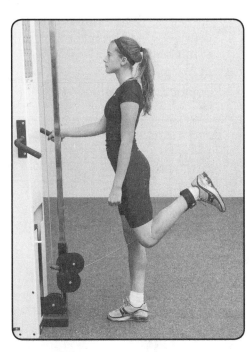

## Straight-Leg Deadlift

Chapter 10 shows how the deadlift helps with the lower back and the glutes, but the simple modification of straightening your legs and either locking or almost locking your knees will virtually eliminate quad help, placing much greater emphasis on the hamstrings Keep in mind though that since the movement bends the waist, the lower back will also get a heavy workout. It is best to use light weight such as small dumbbells while you are learning proper technique. You need to teach the hamstrings how to fire while giving your back a break. When you have the technique down, you can safely add heavier weight.

1. Position the dumbbells or bar in front of you, across your shins (as in the deadlift). Keeping your legs straight (knees locked), bend at the waist and grab the weight.

2. To start the movement, extend at the waist by squeezing your hams and pulling up on the dumbbells. Keep the weight as close as possible to your body, and lift the weight up to waist height. Keep your arms locked at full length during the entire movement.

3. Pause at the top for two counts, and lower the weight back under control. Do not drop the dumbbells.

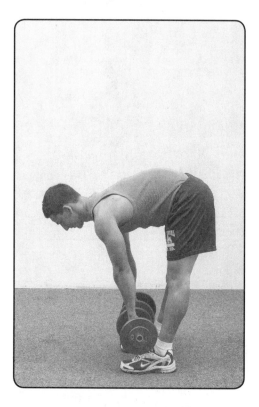 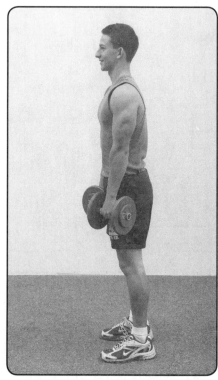

# Stability Ball Leg Curl

This exercise will take your hammys for a ride while forcing your core muscles to maintain a solid posture. Isolating hamstrings is tough, but this exercise is a good candidate, as the position makes it very hard for the glutes to help out. Both your abs and lower back muscles will need to work overtime to keep your torso tight. This exercise is a screamer, but when you get good at it, you will be very happy with both your hamstrings and core development.

1. Lie on your back with your buttocks at the base of a stability ball. Place your legs on top of the ball and dig your heels in. Getting comfortable with the ball takes practice. Try positioning your feet at the far side, and allow your calves to touch while you gain control and balance.
2. Make a bridge by picking your glutes up off the ground. Keep your body straight, legs fully extended, so that your body, the ball, and the floor form a triangle. Your weight will be on your shoulders and heels.
3. Pull the ball toward your butt with your heels by contracting your hamstrings.
4. When fully flexed, hold tight for two counts before letting the ball back out to the starting position.

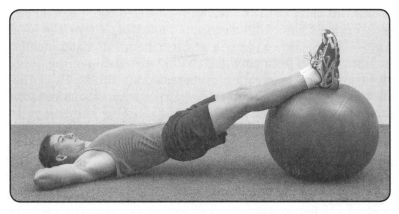

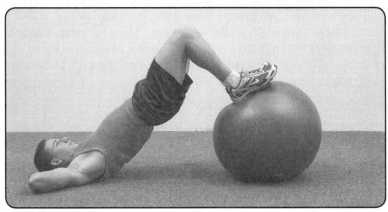

## — TAKE IT TO THE GYM

### Focus on the Hams

In your quest for muscle balance, don't forget to work the hammys. The hamstrings are used during any lift that flexes the knee or extends the hip, such as straight-leg deadlifts, but you cannot assume that your hams get enough work from these exercises. Isolate the hamstrings in order to train them properly. Control your movements, and squeeze at the top of the movement. And don't rush.

The lying leg curl is the best at isolating the hamstrings and preventing strains. It is okay to squeeze your buttocks and pull your hips slightly off the bench when doing leg curls. The most important thing to remember is to use as large a range of motion as possible and squeeze tightly at the contracted position. If you want a real challenge, point your toes. This little modification eliminates the help of the calf muscles and makes the hamstrings work harder.

## — TRAIN AT HOME

### Hit Your Hammys at Home

Hamstrings are tough to isolate without specialized equipment like a leg curl machine. Working them at home means modifying either the straight-leg deadlift or single-leg curl so you can perform them with equipment you have at home. You can also perform the stability ball version of the leg curl. You can perform a straight-leg deadlift using resistance tubing. Place the middle of the tubing under both feet, and extend up the same way as you would with the regular exercise. You will have to grab the tubing low near your ankles and not with the handles so that you can create the proper resistance. For the single-leg curl, you can fix one end of your tubing around your ankle and the other around a solid object on the floor and do your single-leg curl movement.

For a real challenge, you can do a body bridge leg curl (similar to the stability ball leg curl) by lying on your back on a smooth flooring surface. For cushion, place a pillow under your head, and place a towel under your feet so you can slide them. Bridge up onto your shoulders and heels, with your legs almost completely extended. Slide your heels back to your buttocks while maintaining the bridge by squeezing your glutes and hamstrings. Return to the start under control. This is a tough exercise but will yield impressive results with a little practice.

# TRAINING THE HAMSTRINGS

Full range of motion is the key to great-looking hams. Although the best way to isolate the hams is to do leg curls, many exercise combinations will certainly work them well. Definitely do not neglect your hamstrings; they do get a blast on nonspecific exercises, but you need to address them separately. If you are an athlete, it is even more important to make sure your hamstring strength is adequate to reduce the likelihood of injury, so make sure to do at least one hamstring-specific exercise in every leg routine.

| Exercise | Number of reps | Reps per set | Rest between sets |
|---|---|---|---|
| **Routine 1** | | | |
| Lying leg curl | 3 | 10 | 90 sec. |
| Stability ball leg curl | 3 | 10 | 90 sec. |
| **Routine 2** | | | |
| Straight-leg deadlift | 3 | 10 | 2 min. |
| Single-leg curl | 2 each leg | 10 | 90 sec. between same leg |
| **Routine 3** | | | |
| Seated leg curl | 2 | 8 | 90 sec. |
| Lying leg curl | 2 | 8 | 90 sec. |
| Single-leg curl | 1 each leg | 10 | No rest between legs |

# 14

# LOWER LEGS

The muscles on the back of the lower leg are known collectively as the calves. Advanced lifters who have bulked up these muscles call them cows. Two major calf muscles, the gastrocnemius and the soleus, and a host of other muscles help plantar flex the foot (the movement similar to stepping on the gas in your car). The gastrocnemius (the larger muscle) can develop the heart-shaped appearance so highly desired by bodybuilders and is involved in foot and knee actions. The soleus lies under the gastrocnemius. Both muscles can press the foot down strongly and are very important in jumping.

Do not forget the muscles on the front of the lower legs. Although many lifters hardly work them, these muscles are extremely important. Without them, you would not be able to lift your foot upward (dorsiflexion). The main dorsiflexor is the anterior tibialis. These are the muscles that prevent you from tripping over your own feet. Many athletes employ a quick four-way ankle circuit to improve overall ankle stability and help reduce ankle injuries.

## Heel Raise

This exercise is often inaccurately called the calf raise or toe raise. Both names refer to raising the wrong body part. To attack the calves properly, you need to raise your heels off the floor while pivoting on the balls of your feet. The exercise can be done on a machine or on a step. If you use the step, your own body weight probably will be sufficient resistance, but if you want to increase the intensity, pick up a couple of heavy dumbbells and hold them at your sides. For safety, you may need to place a heavy weight plate on the opposite side of the step to ensure it doesn't pop up when you add your weight to the other side.

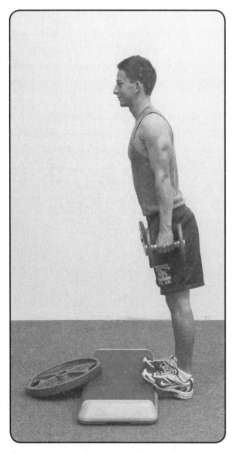

Starting position

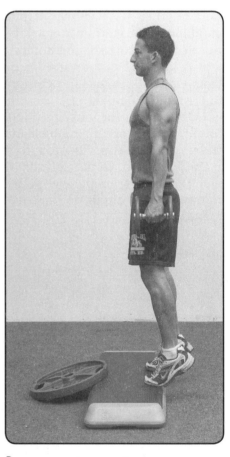

Press up onto your toes

1. Stand with your tiptoes on the edge of the step or machine. The balls of your feet should be secure on the surface, with your heels hanging off the edge.

2. Drive your toes into the ground. Your heels will move up. Pivot on the balls of your feet. Keep pressing your toes until your feet are fully extended. Keep your legs straight during the entire movement; since the gastrocnemius muscle crosses two joints, if the knees bend, the emphasis shifts to the soleus.

3. Hold at the top for two counts before slowly returning to the starting position.

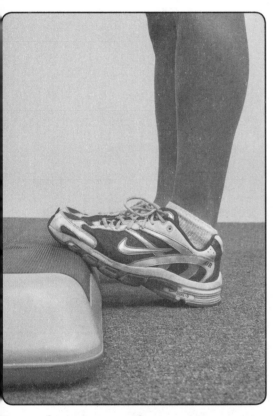

Proper foot alignment for starting position

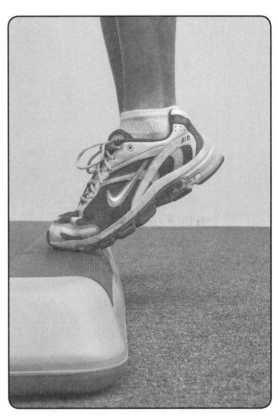

Proper foot alignment for raise

## Leg Press Heel Raise

Take some pressure off your lower back and shoulders by doing a version of the heel raise at a leg press machine.

1. Position yourself in a leg press machine by sitting back and putting your feet on the pad. Instead of placing your feet flat on the pad, hang them off the bottom by placing the balls of your feet against the pad.

2. Perform your heel raise by pushing against the balls of your feet to raise the weight then lowering back down as far as possible. You can leave a slight bend in the knees or extend your legs fully. You may even be able to keep the leg press machine in the safety position during the movement.

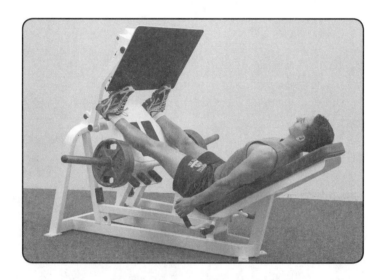

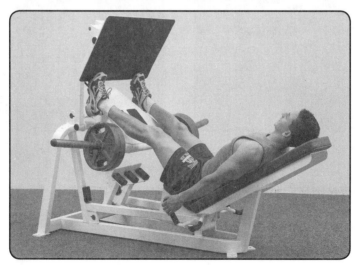

# Single-Leg Heel Raise

Another excellent variation of the heel raise is the single-leg heel raise. This exercise is similar to the heel raise except, to add more resistance, all the weight is on one foot.

1. Stand on the edge of the machine or step with your heel hanging over the edge as in the heel raise. Cross your nonworking leg behind your working leg.
2. Press your toes to lift up your heel.
3. Pause at the top of the movement, squeezing your calf tight. Then, lower back past parallel as deep as possible before beginning the next rep. Try to maximize your range of motion.

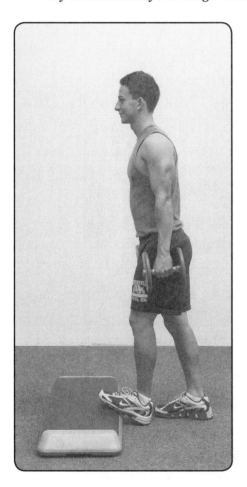 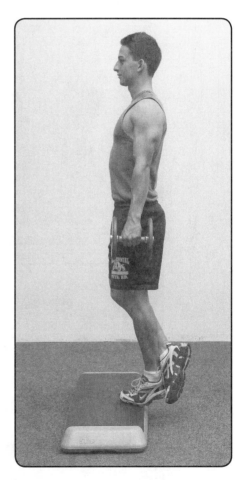

## Seated Calf Heel Raise

The seated calf targets the soleus by removing some of the powerful pulling action of the gastrocnemius. The range of motion for the seated calf is much shorter than for the standing heel raise, although the movement is similar.

1. Sit in the seat of the machine with your knees bent, the resistance on your thighs rather than your shoulders. Place your feet on the foot bar, with your heels hanging over the edge.
2. Press your toes into the foot bar to lift your heels.
3. Pause for two counts at the top of the movement. Then, lower yourself back down under control to your starting position.

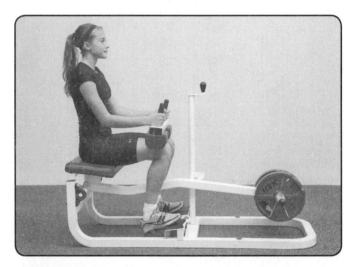

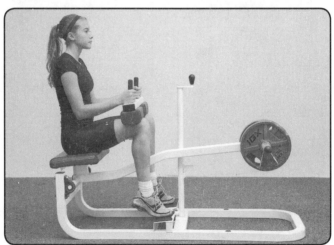

## Squat Heel Raise

Another way to target the calves and mostly the soleus is to get down into a squat position similar to a catcher in baseball. Although the range of motion is short, the burn can be intense and can provide additional strengthening of the support structures of the ankle.

1. Get in the squat position, with feet flat on the floor.
2. Simply roll up onto your tiptoes and hold for two counts, then lower back down.

Both balance and flexibility are needed to perform this exercise, but you can always hold on to something for additional support. At first getting in this position may seem dangerous, but improving your flexibility and strengthening your knees and ankles will prove quite useful later in life.

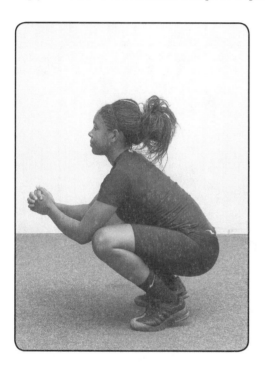 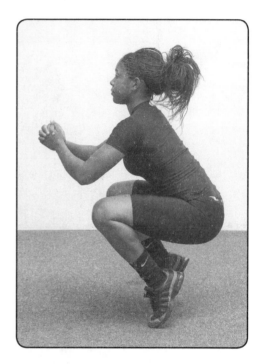

## Toe Pull

Since you will be working your calves, and body balance is so important, working the front of your leg is a must. The toe pull strengthens the front of the lower leg. As its name implies, the motion of the exercise is to pull your toes toward your leg. A few gyms have a toe pull machine, but you can perform toe pulls without a machine by using a partner or tubing.

1. Sit comfortably on a bench with your legs stretched out, your heels hanging over the edge. If you do not have a bench, you can sit on the floor.

2. Point your toes as much as you can, and have your partner grab your toes. (To use tubing, affix one end to an immovable object and the other around your toes.)

3. Flex your feet, pulling against the resistance created by your partner (or the tubing). Do not pull your legs back; instead, concentrate on performing the motion from the ankle joint.

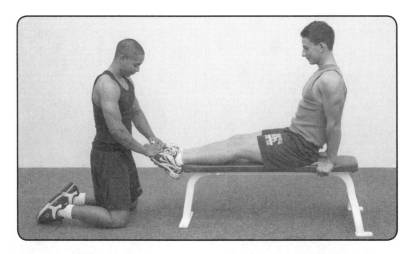

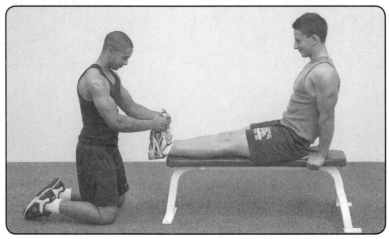

## Ankle Inversion and Eversion

Although preventing ankle rolls in athletics is unlikely, increasing strength will keep the roll from becoming an injury. Turning your feet out (eversion) and in (inversion) under resistance will complete the four-way circuit to strengthen your ankles. Again, remember that strengthening the muscles surrounding the ankle requires that the motion come from the ankle joint.

1. Sit on the floor, and extend your legs out in front. Hook a section of tubing around your foot, or use a partner to create resistance by pushing or pulling in the direction opposite to your movement.

2. Stretch the tubing to the outside of your ankle by placing it around the middle to top of your foot. Pull your foot inward (inversion) by flexing at the ankle; hold for two counts and return.

3. Pull your foot outward (eversion) by flexing at the ankle; hold for two counts and return.

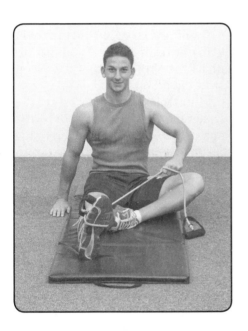 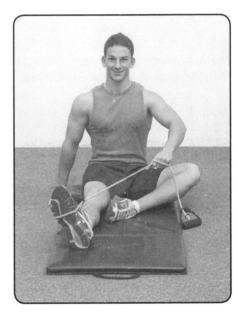

# TAKE IT TO THE GYM

## Developing Heart-Shaped Calves

The key to success in developing your calves is to realize that they work like any other muscle. For some reason, many lifters assume they need to perform hundreds of reps to achieve the desired look, but in reality, the largest contributing factor to shape is genetics. Don't sweat it. Your calves will tone; it may just take some time.

Since these muscles are part of an efficient lever system, they can lift considerably more weight than an exercise such as a biceps curl. Even though the calf muscles are not that big, their anatomical mechanics (how they are positioned on your leg) make them strong and thus difficult to train effectively. Use heavier weight, but perform the same number of reps as you would for any other body part. Use the full range of motion, and perform each rep under control. Work the muscle in a smooth action from start to finish. Do not jerk your heels upward. That is a no-no. Muscles work best when they are continuously stressed through the entire range of motion.

Calf muscles are easily strained, so before training your calves, warm them up and stretch them out. If they feel tight, do not train them. If you plan to perform long-duration aerobic activity such as running later that day or on the following day, work the calves lightly or not at all.

Anecdotal evidence suggests that foot position variations may target the inner and outer portions of the gastrocnemius more effectively. Currently, these theories have not been proven conclusively. Feel free, however, to try pointing your toes in to work the outer head or pointing your toes out to work the inner head.

# TRAIN AT HOME

## Work Your Calves on Your Couch

Considering the fact that couch lounging has created a society of overweight people, it is nice to know that you can actually improve your strength while watching TV. Almost all of the exercises in this chapter can be performed at home using resistance tubing or a training partner. But here is a simple way to catch up on your local news and build better-looking calves. While sitting upright with your feet on the floor, place a couple of books under your toes and press down on your knees (or if you have kids, have them sit on your lap) to create resistance. Then perform a seated heel raise as you normally would. Unless you can create enough resistance, this move will not be as effective as hitting the gym, but it is certainly more enjoyable.

# TONING THE CALVES

You can work the calves in two ways: with legs extended or legs flexed. How you choose to get to that position is up to you. As long as you can create enough resistance, it is recommended to work the calves in both ways during each workout. If you are short on time, use one way for one workout, then the other way for the next workout, alternating every other workout.

Generally, size is the goal for most lifters. For hypertrophy, go for 12 reps with no more than 90 seconds of rest between sets (60 seconds is preferred). If you can, perform another set for a total of three sets in all.

| Exercise | Number of sets | Reps per set | Rest between sets |
|---|---|---|---|
| **Routine 1** | | | |
| Heel raise | 2 | 12 | 90 sec. |
| Seated calf heel raise | 2 | 12 | 90 sec. |
| Toe pull | 3 | 12 | 60 sec. |
| **Routine 2** | | | |
| Heel raise | 2 | 10 | 90 sec. |
| Toe pull | 2 | 10 | 60 sec. |
| Ankle inversion | 2 each foot | 10 | 60 sec. |
| Ankle eversion | 2 each foot | 10 | 60 sec. |
| **Routine 3** | | | |
| Squat heel raise | 2 | 12 | 90 sec. |
| Leg press heel raise | 2 | 12 | 90 sec. |
| Ankle inversion | 2 each foot | 12 | 60 sec. |
| Ankle eversion | 2 each foot | 12 | 60 sec. |

# 15

# PROGRAM DESIGN

If you have tried a weight training program in the past, you may have watched someone in a gym or asked for guidance from someone you hoped had a good idea of what to do. Most likely you were told to do three sets of 10 reps of a basic set of exercises using machines if you were a beginner or free weights if you were more advanced. Thirty years ago, this method of programming was the backbone of the traditional resistance program. However, over the last decade or so, the world of weight training has changed dramatically. The field of resistance training is now surrounded by an entire industry filled with gimmicks purporting tremendous gains. This industry also includes numerous self-proclaimed experts who have their own prescriptions for what works best in the weight room. Equally confusing is the mess of contradicting scientific evidence explaining what does and doesn't work. The result is that the average weightlifter is left with many questions: How much weight should I use, and how many reps and sets should I perform? Does exercise order matter? Why are some exercises better than others?

Amid the commercial hype and the enshrined lifting rituals (which may be based more on tradition than science) exists a limited number of well-designed research studies that have examined the previous questions with scrutiny and credibility. From these studies we have learned that muscles must be challenged and that the best long-term adaptations occur when a regular program is followed and all muscle groups are addressed. Further, specific adaptations are achieved when muscles are given specific exercises with varying loads and both high and low repetition schemes. Higher reps (15 plus) develop endurance, moderate reps (8 to 12) develop overall size, and lower reps (3 to 8) develop power and strength. And finally, rest is needed to see effort pay off.

Certainly, specific exercises help achieve specific results, but the ideal combination and total volume (total amount of work done measured by sets × reps) for an entire workout is unknown. With so many new exercises being developed, it is hard to decide which ones to use. However, it appears there is no right or wrong way to work out as long as you adhere to proper technique and form. This may seem frustrating if you are looking for a black-and-white solution, but the shades of gray keep practitioners and researchers on their toes as they continue to provide new challenges for those engaging in exercise. One clear answer is that there are no shortcuts; hard work is the key to success.

# METHODS FOR CREATING TRAINING PROGRAMS

The decision to start a weight training program is based on an end goal. So training without purpose is like looking for buried treasure without a map—your likelihood of success is slim. Since each person has a unique goal and since adaptation is specific to the stress, there are several methods of constructing a workout program. Each training method has different set, rep, and resistance variations. If you follow the overload principle, you must make sure that the resistance becomes difficult by the last one or two reps of each set. No matter how many reps are required, the resistance should be challenging once you are familiar with the exercise. If you use weights that are too light, it will take longer to see results. If you use weights that are too heavy, you risk burnout, overtraining, and injury.

## Training for Muscular Endurance

To gain muscular endurance, you have two choices. You can either extend the set by completing more repetitions or rest for a shorter amount of time between sets. Generally, a set of 12 to 20 reps should last at least 30 seconds but not more than 90 seconds. A prolonged set will encourage lactic acid buildup. This causes that familiar burning sensation and ultimately leads to fatigue. Although lactic acid buildup tends to get a bad rap, if you learn to push through the burn and tolerate the pain, your body will become more accustomed to handling it and further build your muscle's endurance capacity. So the next time you feel the burn, go for a few more reps.

Aim for one to three sets of 15 to 25 repetitions, resting for 30 to 60 seconds between sets. Another alternative is to perform three to five sets of 10 to 15 reps, resting for 15 to 30 seconds between sets.

## Training for Muscular Strength

If strength is your goal, you need to use relatively heavy resistance to perform fewer repetitions per set, and you'll need to rest for two to three minutes between sets. The goal of this type of training is to increase the overall strength of a muscle or group of muscles. Strength training usually includes exercises that work the major muscle groups, such as the bench press, seated row, and squat. The catalyst for strength gain, however, is not the number of reps but how hard you work in the lower rep range. If you can easily get 6 to 8 reps and choose to stop, you will not build strength effectively. Neither will you help your strength efforts if the weight is too light and you do more reps. Your last few reps should stop you dead in your tracks and either require a spot to get another rep or force you to stop completely.

For best results, perform one to three sets of 6 to 8 repetitions, resting for two and a half to three minutes between sets.

## Training for Muscular Size

Most people who work out want to improve their overall appearance. For men, increasing muscle size is usually the number one goal. Women usually want to become leaner or more toned. Whatever your goal, the results you want take time, and in all cases, size and muscle density are necessary if you wish to have a figure with muscle definition.

Hypertrophy is the technical term for building size, increasing mass, or bodybuilding. Despite popular myth, using very heavy weight as in strength training does not promote size increases as rapidly. Hypertrophy training falls somewhere between strength and endurance training. Training for hypertrophy involves a moderate number of reps with moderate to heavy weight and average rest periods. For those of you afraid to build size rapidly, especially women, don't worry—a few weeks or even months of hypertrophy training will increase muscle size, but getting tree trunk legs and boulder-sized biceps takes many years. Instead, if you are working out to see some definition, to get a few "cuts" in your arms, or to look good at the beach, this is the strategy for you.

The optimal way to increase size is to perform one to three sets of 8 to 12 repetitions (usually 10 to 12), resting for 90 seconds between sets.

## Training for Power

Power training is explosive in nature and requires very quick movements using as much weight as possible while still lifting explosively. The advantage of explosive training for sport, although still under investigation, appears to be substantial in athletes playing sports where explosive contact is a regular part of the game. Contact sports such as football have seen some of the best improvements. However, because of the inherent risk, the average person who is looking to get in shape, tone up, and look good probably need not spend time doing explosive lifting. Only skilled lifters and sport-specific athletes should engage in power training.

If you are considering performing explosive movements, use your own body weight, and make sure someone keeps an eye on your form. For true power development, use light to moderate weight for three to five sets of 3 to 5 reps, lifted as explosively as possible.

# TYPES OF ROUTINES

To add variety and challenge to your basic program, try a few of the following modifications. Just as you can choose from different exercises and modes of resistance, you can choose from several different ways to train. Use the guidelines described in this section to determine reps and sets, the type of weight used, and the order of exercises. These are some of the more popular training methods.

## Supersets and Multisets

If you want an efficient workout that provides maximum benefit in minimum time, this is the method for you. In a superset, you perform two exercises one after the other, with little or no rest in between. This method has a distinct advantage in reducing overall exercise time and increasing muscle size, although it is not recommended if your primary goal is to develop strength.

Complete the first set of the first exercise, then move on to the next exercise without resting. The second exercise should work the opposite muscle group. For example, for a leg superset, begin with leg extensions, and then move on to lying leg curls with no rest between sets. Essentially, you recover from the first exercise during the second exercise, although this recovery is not complete.

A multiset joins three or more exercises. For example, an arm multiset might include triceps push-downs, dumbbell curls, and lateral raises. The longer you continue without rest, the more likely you will fatigue. If you are performing more than one superset or multiset, rest for one to two minutes before beginning the next superset or multiset. Here are some popular superset groups:

- Leg superset: leg extension, lying leg curl
- Upper arm superset: supine triceps extension, dumbbell curl
- Upper back and shoulder superset: shoulder press, lat pull-down
- Upper back and chest superset: bench press, seated row

For each exercise, try two or three sets of 10 to 12 reps. For example, for the leg superset, perform a set of 10 to 12 leg extensions followed by a set of 10 to 12 lying leg curls, with no rest between exercises. Rest briefly before beginning the second set of leg extensions.

If you want some challenging multisets, check out the triple exhaust routine in chapter 16.

## Circuit Training

Circuit training extends the multiset idea. All the exercises in a particular circuit follow one another with little rest. If you want to perform more than one circuit, rest three to five minutes between circuits. Circuits decrease time spent in the gym and increase muscular endurance. Hypertrophy will occur over time. You can alternate between upper and lower body exercises or between front and back exercises or both. See chapter 16 for some great sample circuits, or you can create your own.

## Preexhaust Training

As the name implies, in preexhaust training, the lifter forces a muscle or group of muscles to become exhausted before moving on to another exercise that works the same muscle. Preexhaust training adds variety and challenge to a routine. Begin with an isolated single-joint exercise, then perform a double- or multijoint movement that works the same muscle group. Smaller muscles usually fatigue before larger ones, so the larger muscles in the multijoint movement are not entirely worked. The fatiguing smaller muscles usually cause the set to end early.

Although it can seem confusing, preexhaust training makes a lot of sense. Let's look at an example. Consider the typical weekend warrior or bodybuilder who begins his chest routine with the bench press. Pecs are the major muscle group involved, but the triceps and front deltoids are worked as well. Since the weakest links in the bench press are the deltoids and triceps, they usually fatigue first. The weaker muscles lose their force capability, causing the set to end before the pecs have had a chance to break down completely. The net result is that the pecs don't reach complete exhaustion and require further concentrated exercises. So our warrior moves on to pec flys, cable crosses, or another pec exercise, but he can't seem to get that maximum burn.

The solution is preexhaust training, and here's how it can be implemented in the example. Let's use the same exercises (bench press and pec fly) but reverse the order and superset them. In other words, we preexhaust the pecs with a pec fly set to failure, then immediately follow it with a bench press. When our warrior finishes the set, his pecs should be adequately exhausted. Also, as he continues through the rest of his workout using preexhaust training, he will find his delts and triceps don't limit his pec workout. All three muscle groups receive an equal amount of work.

Another variation of preexhaust training is to complete all sets of the preexhaust isolated single-joint exercise before moving on to the multijoint exercise and completing its sets separately rather than supersetting them. Both methods of preexhaust training are effective, but doing both variations in a workout creates even more variety. Here are some of the most popular combinations:

- Chest: dumbbell pec fly followed by bench press
- Upper back: dumbbell pullover followed by lat pull-down
- Shoulders and upper arms: supine triceps extension followed by shoulder press

## Postexhaust Training

Postexhaust training is similar to preexhaust training except that the exhaustive movement follows the initial movement. A postexhaust exercise is usually a single-joint movement that isolates a particular muscle group. This movement follows a multijoint or main core movement.

The rationale behind this method of training is threefold. First, performing a postexhaust exercise immediately after a major movement increases the likelihood of overloading that particular muscle group, especially if a smaller stabilizer muscle limits maximal performance, as in the bench press example. Second, postexhaust training increases the ability to isolate a muscle or muscle group that needs the extra work, especially if it is hard to train or develop. Third, postexhaust exercises are a form of conditioning because the length of a normal set is extended by 30 seconds or more. This makes it a valuable method for muscular endurance training. Here are some of the most popular combinations:

- Chest: bench press followed by dumbbell pec fly
- Upper back: lat pull-down followed by dumbbell pullover
- Legs: leg press followed by leg extension

## Drop Sets

The *drop* in drop sets, also known as strip sets or burn sets, refers to the act of decreasing resistance. A drop set is performed as an extension of the initial set of an exercise. During the drop, resistance is removed by removing plates in free weight exercises or lowering the weight in machine exercises. The lifter completes a prescribed number of reps to a point of relative failure, the weight is immediately decreased, and the lifter continues for another set of reps until failure. The number of drops varies depending on the goal of the exercise and the lifter's ability to tolerate the pain. The drop should be about 20 percent of the initial weight each time, but it varies depending on the lifter's tolerance.

Popular drop exercises are bench presses, rows, triceps exercises, biceps exercises, and leg extensions. For example, if you started with 150 pounds (70 kg) for a bench press, you might perform one set of 8 reps with the 150 pounds, then drop to 120 pounds (55 kg), then to 90 pounds (40 kg), and finally to 60 pounds (30 kg). With the 120 pounds and each subsequent drop, you should expect to do no more than four or five reps and possibly only one or two.

## Negative Training

Negative training emphasizes the eccentric portion (when the muscle lengthens) of the lift. The advantage of negative training is that the lifter can use more weight, causing the body to adapt to the increase in weight. The disadvantage is that it increases the risk of injury and requires a spotter. Negative training can be done with free weights or machines.

Negative training can be performed in two ways. In the first way, the lifter does a normal set until fatigued, then finishes with negative sets. To do this, you would have your spotter help with the positive, or concentric, portion of the lift, then you would lower the weight (the negative portion of the lift) slowly under control. This method works well because a person is as much as 20 to 40 percent stronger in the eccentric phase. The concentric movement will cause fatigue before the eccentric movement. Therefore, to achieve a good eccentrically fatigued state, the negative portion can be worked for additional reps while the spotter helps the lifter during the concentric portion of the exercise. Exercises such as bench presses and shoulder presses, leg extensions and leg curls, and most pulls work well with this type of routine.

The second way to train is called negative emphasized. As the name implies, the rep is normal except that the negative portion is exaggerated by increasing the time the lifter takes to lower the weight. Emphasized negatives are the most popular, safest, and most productive exercises of the two because they are controlled by the lifter. In a negative rep, it should take at least five seconds to lower the weight. Any faster and the lifter is not truly working against the weight to slow it down.

For negatives to work properly, the lifter needs to exert maximal force against the weight (just as when pushing it up) to slow the weight down; otherwise it will drop like a rock, and the negative will be ineffective. If the amount of weight is correct, the lifter's maximal effort will still cause the weight to descend. If the weight is too heavy, the lifter's effort against it will not last long enough to create a benefit, or the weight will just drop. If the weight is too light, the lifter will take too long to lower it and may not exert enough force. Too light a weight is not as bad as too heavy a weight.

No matter which method of negative training you use, the result will be greater development from a single set and greater fatigue from eccentric exercise. The most popular exercises for negative training are the machine bench press, dumbbell curl, and leg extension.

## Forced Repetitions to Exhaustion

For forced repetitions, the lifter is forced to complete more reps than she can complete on her own. A spotter assists the lifter in performing the forced reps, but the spotter provides only a little help. If the spotter needs to help a lot, then the weight is too heavy or the set is over. Forced reps are crucial for developing ultimate strength. This method also prevents cheating and keeps the emphasis of the exercise and the tension on the specific muscle or muscle group. Some good exercises for forced reps are the bench press, supine triceps extension, dumbbell curl, leg extension, and lying leg curl. Avoid forced reps with very technical lifts such as the squat and lunge.

## Slow Training

Slow training is good for developing both hypertrophy and muscular endurance. There are several versions of slow training. In one version, known as super slow training, the exercise is performed at a very slow pace, taking 30 to 60 seconds to complete a single repetition. This method is difficult to perform and often boring. Although advocates of super slow training believe it is a good method, there is little evidence to support this theory.

Other methods of slow training provide both a strong stimulus for improvement and a great challenge. A great method of slow training is to use a 5-second concentric phase followed by a 5- to 10-second eccentric phase of a single repetition. You can further enhance slow training by adding an isometric hold at the end of the concentric movement. Taking a leg curl as an example, perform a 5-second concentric contraction, hold for 5 seconds at the top of the movement (fully contracted), then perform a 5-second eccentric movement. Multiple reps can be performed (usually five).

## Pyramid System

There are three versions of this training, with three kinds of pyramids, giving rise to nine different pyramid combinations. Figure 15.1 illustrates the possible pyramid scenarios. To pyramid up, you can increase the weight and decrease the reps, increase the reps and decrease the weight, or increase both weight and reps. To pyramid down, decrease weight and increase reps, decrease reps and increase weight, or decrease both. For a real challenge, try pyramiding up and down. This can be done one of three ways: increase weight and decrease reps up, then decrease weight and increase reps down; increase reps and decrease weight up, then decrease reps and increase weight down; or increase both weight and reps up, then decrease both down.

A good pyramid ensures that the lifter will get strength, size, and endurance benefits as well as fully exhausted muscles if performed with the right amount of weight and rest. The major drawback with a pyramid is that the lifter has to save strength for later sets and therefore, if the weight is not properly dialed in, may never get in a truly good set.

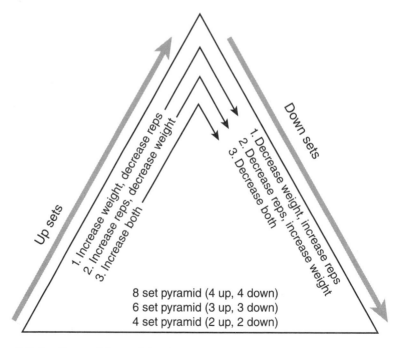

**Figure 15.1**  Pyramid combinations.

## Concentration (or Blitz) System

In the concentration, or blitz, system, the entire workout concentrates on a specific body part or movement. Sometimes as many as 6 sets are performed for each exercise and as many as 30 sets for the body part. For bodybuilders, this type of routine helps them focus on a weaker or smaller part that needs development. However, muscle group or body part concentration is not going to benefit an athlete training for sport performance. Training a specific movement or exercise may have merit if constant repetition of the same movement occurs during play. Concentration training typically requires several sessions per week to train the entire body and thus is not practical for the general population. Remember, this is truly hard-core training. Extreme muscle soreness will occur in most people. Here is a sample blitz training routine:

- Straight bar curls: $6 \times 12$
- Isolated dumbbell curls: $6 \times 12$ each arm
- Preacher curls: $6 \times 12$
- Cable curls: $6 \times 12$

## Split Training

Almost all training, except for a full-body workout, uses some form of split training. In split training, certain muscles, muscle groups, or body parts become the focus. This method is effective if your schedule allows a few more sessions per week in the weight room. If you split a workout for the upper body from a workout for the lower body and perform each on separate days, you create a split routine.

You can take it a step further and split upper body exercises or lower body exercises. For example, you may work the chest, triceps, and shoulders one day and the back and biceps another day. Another variation of the split routine is to split your workout into morning and evening sessions, perhaps working the lower body in the morning and the upper body in the evening. This can be effective if you have other demands on your time. Advanced lifters perform even more elaborate splits.

Whatever type of split you use, make your routines time effective and goal specific. Here are some common split routines:

- Upper body/lower body
- Chest, triceps, shoulders/back and biceps/legs

## Push and Pull

Push–pull training incorporates split training, supersetting, or both. You may train push movements one day and pull the next day, or train both push and pull movements on the same day by alternating in the form of a superset or by resting between sets. On the other hand, if time is an issue and you want to create muscular balance, you could complete an entire push exercise for

| Exercise | Number of sets | Reps per set | Rest between sets |
|---|---|---|---|
| **Push–pull 1** | | | |
| Bench press | 2 | 10 | 90 sec. |
| Seated row | 2 | 10 | 90 sec. |
| Shoulder press | 2 | 10 | 90 sec. |
| Lat pull-down | 2 | 10 | 90 sec. |
| Triceps push-down | 2 | 10 | 90 sec. |
| Dumbbell curl | 2 | 10 | 90 sec. |
| **Push–pull 2** | | | |
| Circuit | 2-3 circuits | | 3 min. between circuits |
| Bench press | 1 | 10 | 60 sec. |
| Seated row | 1 | 10 | 60 sec. |
| Shoulder press | 1 | 10 | 60 sec. |
| Lat pull-down | 1 | 10 | 60 sec. |
| Triceps push-down | 1 | 10 | 60 sec. |
| Dumbbell curl | 1 | 10 | 60 sec. |

all its prescribed sets before moving on to the pull exercise or vice versa. For example, a lifter may do three sets of bench presses followed by three sets of seated rows. The advantage of a push–pull routine is that both sides of a body part get worked, resulting in symmetry and balance between front and back. Often lifters spend too much time working specific muscles and forget about the importance of muscle balance for avoiding injury.

# PUTTING YOUR PROGRAM TOGETHER

So, what should you do? The answer lies in the type of training program you want and the quality you are looking for. Each training method requires different variations with respect to sets, reps, and resistance. The fact that there are so many different training methods is ample proof that a training program is unique to the lifter. The key to figuring out what is best for you is to practice, using the principles discussed in this chapter and in chapters 1 through 4. Work hard and use proper technique. The results you achieve are a function of the quality of the repetition and the degree of adaptation in your muscles. You can achieve your desired results by manipulating the number of sets and reps and the amount of rest. If you are properly following the overload principle, the resistance should become difficult by the last one or two reps of the set.

Recall from chapter 3 the importance of performing the perfect repetition. So no matter which exercise you choose and which program method you follow, every rep needs to be perfectly repeated for the entire set. When you can successfully complete all the reps and sets of a particular exercise, only then is it time to increase the weight for your next workout.

You can choose from several hundred exercises with various modifications. With each exercise, you can use a machine, free weights, dumbbells, resistance tubing, or other form of resistance. In addition, each machine may vary in speed or leverage based on its cam or computer system. Each form of resistance has its advantages and disadvantages (see the table on page 18). Whichever mode you choose, make sure the exercise is specific to what you are trying to achieve and each rep is as perfect as possible.

Deciding which type of training program to use may be challenging. Your goals undoubtedly will change in time or even soon after you begin working out. Understanding the contents of this book and how to perform different exercises gives you the tools to keep up with your constantly changing life. Perhaps time is on your side now, and you have plenty of time to work out. At some point you will be very short on time and need to make changes. You may want to increase size today but build better muscle endurance in the future. The great thing about weight training is that you can continually make changes. You can add mini challenges to push yourself to reach your goals, surpass them, and make new ones.

Program design is something even the best coaches in the world continually challenge. If you put 20 coaches in a room and ask them to develop a program for soccer players, you will get 20 different programs. Each person has a unique perspective, and with that comes a unique stamp of approval. Choose your exercises and develop your program based on your goals. Draw yourself a map of where you are and where you want to be, and write yourself a set of directions by creating the perfect workout—for you! You can also follow our basic programs presented in chapter 16, but by all means make changes so that you see results.

If after 4 weeks you see no change in strength, size, endurance, or general health, take a gut check and make sure you have been working hard; if so, you need to reevaluate your program and make changes. You now understand how many reps you need for a particular outcome. You now understand the importance of rest. And you now have hundreds of variations of exercises from which to choose. Follow the simple rules of progression and overload, create variety, and respect rest. If you work hard every set, your goals will be reached.

# PERIODIZATION IS NOT JUST FOR ATHLETES

Generally after 8 weeks (although some find that even 12 or more weeks of the same exercises is beneficial), your muscles will be screaming for change, either from boredom or overuse. In advanced lifters, usually 4 or 5 weeks is all the body can handle before change is required. In some cases injury or overtraining occurs, but for most, the gains reach a plateau and slow considerably, stop, or even reverse. The method of changing routines is part of the basis of periodization, a term that describes how exercise is prescribed over a longer training cycle.

An in-depth discussion of periodization is beyond the scope of this book, but a quick understanding of the concept may help your training for the rest of your life. Periodization is based on an idea from a medical doctor in the 1920s who was trying to combat disease. He found that after stress, the body goes into a rebuilding phase and gets stronger. Over time, the body adapts and prepares for the next stress. Called the general adaptation theory, this suggests that cells undergo changes when stressed; if you continue stressing the system and changing the stress, the body continues to adapt. Since muscles are cells, this is also the basis for how muscle grows and develops. Every time we work out, we stress our muscles, forcing them to respond by adapting by either increasing size, strength, speed, flexibility, endurance, or all of these factors. But over time and regular training, the program will eventually become stale and the body may become overtrained or even injured. Thus the idea behind periodization is to prevent that staleness, reduce overtraining, and continue to make gains to keep the body healthy.

The principle of periodization is to systematically make small changes by altering some or all of the following factors: the number of sets, number of reps, length of rest, frequency of workouts, and types of exercises. The key word is *systematically*, although it is nearly impossible for a beginner to predict how the body will respond and what changes will be necessary. Seasoned trainers and strength coaches, however, can do this with some degree of certainty based on their past experiences, and thus a college football strength coach has a good idea of how his players will progress over their four-year playing career. For you, the beginner, or even advanced lifter, this means that when you feel as if things are boring, you notice you are not making gains, or you simply think it is time to change things up, do so! Keep track of your changes, and over time you too will become good at predicting training cycles.

In its basic form, periodization means shifting workouts from endurance to strength or hypertrophy and from hypertrophy to strength or power. In fact, there are endless combinations, but generally a periodized program looks at a full year of training (called a macrocycle) and builds smaller programs within (known as mesocycles and microcycles) that change every 4 to 12 weeks. For athletes, the meso- and microcycles may be structured by the particular demands of the sports season. For others, the cycles may vary based on school years, vacations, sickness, and anything that would disrupt normal daily routine for more then a few days.

There is no need to get complicated, but before starting your training routine, you should consider your long-term goals. Perhaps you will find that a strength program is a good start, but endurance or size training may be something you will want later on. When you feel your body wanting something else, that is the time to make the change. To learn more about implementing periodization in your training, see *Designing Resistance Training Programs, Third Edition* by Steven Fleck and William Kraemer. For the time being, consider developing a training program that changes within 4 to 8 weeks, and see how your progress continues—and how much better you feel when you stick to your weight training program because it continues to challenge and reward you.

# 16

# SAMPLE PROGRAMS

Choosing the correct sequence of exercises, the number of sets and reps, and how much weight is only one part of successful weight training. Being dedicated and pushing yourself to reach and exceed your potential are other essential factors for success. Without them, you are spinning your wheels. But remember, too, that working hard does not have to mean boring. You can have fun with your program. In fact, you need to if you want to make exercise a regular part of your daily life.

In the beginning, it is important to exercise at least three times per week to get your engine started and to make weight training a habit. Do yourself and your body a favor by finding the time to work out, even if you can squeeze in only a few minutes. Unfortunately, there is no way to get around working hard, but you can have periods when you don't do as much or reduce your intensity, such as during holidays, breaks, or just a general need for a rest. Once you have been training for a while, maintenance plans are sufficient, and thus you can reduce the number of times you exercise and still reap the rewards. When you can reduce your efforts and go to a maintenance phase is still under debate scientifically, but the general rule is that you need to be working hard for several months before considering dropping off for anything more than a few days or a week. There is no better feeling than the strength and confidence you will gain. The world is your oyster—so go get that pearl and reach your potential!

The following programs are meant to be challenging. Adjust the weights accordingly, and track your results so you can measure your success. Feel free to modify any workout to meet your needs. A good workout design is one that helps you obtain your goals. Don't be afraid to go against convention and hit a few extra sets of arm curls if bulgier biceps are your thing. If a program has a barbell bench press and you only have dumbbells, make the substitution and move on. But most important, keep safety in mind. More is not better; only better is better. And remember, the harder you work, the sorer you may become, so don't overdo it. Otherwise, you may not be able to raise your arms overhead the next day.

# OVERALL BODY WORKOUT

For most people, a total-body workout is the best choice. If you have a full schedule or do other physical activity, then this type of workout is for you. A total-body workout should take 30 to 60 minutes to complete. If you perform only one set per exercise, it may take less time. Remember, perform a good warm-up and stretch before beginning the workout. The more generalized your workout, the longer it will take for those individual muscles to make gains. When you hit a full-body workout, you do not zero in on individual parts but on your body as a whole, which improves overall fitness and strength. You should lift weights before other activity such as aerobics if your primary goal is to improve muscle strength and size. For general health, however, it doesn't matter which you do first.

## General Workout

This is the standard workout that most health club and general fitness enthusiasts advocate. It is a great starter workout that covers all the basics to get you up and running and improve overall health and fitness.

| Exercise | Sets | Reps | Rest |
| --- | --- | --- | --- |
| Bench press | 2 | 12 | 60-90 sec. |
| Machine pec fly | 2 | 12 | 60-90 sec. |
| Shoulder press | 2 | 12 | 60-90 sec. |
| Seated row | 2 | 12 | 60-90 sec. |
| Triceps push-down | 2 | 12 | 60-90 sec. |
| Dumbbell curl | 2 | 12 | 60-90 sec. |
| Leg press | 2 | 12 | 60-90 sec. |
| Leg extension | 2 | 12 | 60-90 sec. |
| Lying leg curl | 2 | 12 | 60-90 sec. |
| Heel raise | 2 | 12 | 60-90 sec. |

## Total-Body Supercircuit

Perform one set of 12 repetitions for each of the exercises in these circuits. Perform the exercises in order, with minimal rest between them—only enough to set up the next machine. You may choose to perform any one of the three circuits. When the circuit is complete, take a breather for about two minutes, and then attempt a second circuit. If you feel especially good, try a third circuit. If you choose to do more than one circuit on a particular day, go through each circuit only once.

| Circuit 1<br>Perform 12 reps per exercise | Circuit 2<br>Perform 12 reps per exercise | Circuit 3<br>Perform 12 reps per exercise |
|---|---|---|
| Bench press | Bench press | Lunge |
| Leg press | Seated row | Incline bench press |
| Seated row | Shoulder press | Leg press |
| Lying leg curl | Dumbbell curl | Lat pull-down |
| Shoulder press | Triceps push-down | Single-leg curl |
| Leg extension | Leg press | Lateral raise |
| Triceps push-down | Seated leg curl | Heel raise |
| Heel raise | Leg extension | Supine triceps extension |
| Dumbbell curl | Heel raise | Toe pull |
| Seated calf heel raise | Seated calf heel raise | Dumbbell curl |
| Crunch | Crunch | Ab circuit (15 reps each exercise):<br>Crunch<br>Twisting crunch (each side)<br>Pelvic raise |
| Back extension | Back extension | |
| Rest about 2 min. | Rest about 2 min. | Rest about 2 min. |

# Resistance Training 101 and 102

Another great way to target the total body is to use a combination of machine and free weight exercises. We call this the basics, so keep in mind the emphasis should be placed on technique, not weight lifted, and sets should not be taken to muscular failure. Alternate between workout 1 and workout 2, and allow at least 48 to 72 hours of rest between workouts.

| Workout 1<br>Complete 15 reps per set<br>Rest 90-120 sec. between sets | | Workout 2<br>Complete 15 reps per set<br>Rest 90-120 sec. between sets | |
|---|---|---|---|
| Exercise | Number<br>of sets | Exercise | Number<br>of sets |
| Dumbbell squat | 3 | Leg press | 3 |
| Machine seated row | 3 | Lat pull-down | 3 |
| Machine bench press | 3 | Modified push-up | 3 |
| Dumbbell shoulder press | 2 | Lateral raise | 2 |
| Dumbbell curl | 2 | Cable curl | 2 |
| Triceps push-down | 2 | Dumbbell triceps kickback | 2 |
| Crunch | 2 | Twisting crunch | 2 |
| Superman | 2 | Superman (opposite arm and leg) | 2 |

# Body-Weight Circuits

Body-weight circuits are great when you need to work out at home or just need a change from the gym. Don't use having kids as an excuse not to work out. If you're a parent, your children can do this workout with you. Each exercise within the circuit can be performed for repetitions or time. Beginners should start with approximately 12 to 15 reps per exercise or as many reps as can be performed in 30 seconds. To increase the intensity of the workouts, perform more reps, increase the duration of each set within the circuit, or perform multiple circuits with little to no rest in between.

| Beginner circuit<br>12-15 reps per exercise | Intermediate circuit<br>15-20 reps per exercise | Advanced circuit<br>20 or more reps per exercise |
|---|---|---|
| Squat | Walking lunge | Single-leg squat |
| Superman | Squat | Walking lunge |
| Modified push-up | Modified push-up | Squat |
| Bench dip | Bench dip | Wide-hand push-up |
| Crunch | Plank | Close-hand push-up |
| Plank | Crunch | Lateral plank raise |
| Jumping jacks (30 sec.) | Superman | Crunch |

# Fitness Enthusiast Workout

If you're looking to step it up a little, this routine is for you. It's perfect for anyone looking to push a little harder while getting it all done on the same day. Perform this routine three times per week. Try sticking with the exercise order prescribed to maximize your gains.

| Day 1<br>6-10 reps per set<br>Rest 1-2 min. between sets | | Day 2<br>>8-12 reps per set<br>Rest 1-2 min. between sets | | Day 3<br>12-15 reps per set<br>Rest 1-2 min. between sets | |
|---|---|---|---|---|---|
| Exercise | Sets | Exercise | Sets | Exercise | Sets |
| Squat | 3 | Walking lunge | 3 | Leg press | 3 |
| Lying leg curl | 2 | Seated leg curl | 2 | Single-leg heel raise | 2 |
| Seated calf heel raise | 2 | Heel raise | 2 | Lying leg curl | 2 |
| Bench press | 3 | Machine bench press | 3 | Dumbbell incline bench press | 3 |
| Dumbbell row | 3 | Lat pull-down | 3 | Cable seated row | 3 |
| Dumbbell shoulder press | 2 | Alternating front raise | 2 | Lateral raise | 2 |
| V-bar triceps push-down<br>E-Z bar curl | 2<br>supersets | Supine triceps extension<br>Dumbbell curl | 2<br>supersets | Dumbbell triceps kickback<br>Hammer curl | 2<br>supersets |
| Crunch<br>Superman (opposite arm and leg) | 3<br>supersets | Crunch<br>Pelvic raise | 3<br>supersets | Crunch<br>Superman | 3<br>supersets |

# Great Pyramid

Using the pyramid technique, this workout hits all rep range, rest interval, and weight combinations. The trick is to manage your sets, reps, and weights so that you maximize recovery. This workout can be added to a standard whole-body training program in place of one workout per week or can be performed for a week or so just for a change of pace. Beginner and intermediate trainees should pyramid up (set one through set three for beginners or set one through set four for intermediate lifters). Advanced lifters can perform one or two full pyramids (which contain three sets up and three sets down) when going up and down, or as many as four pyramids (three sets up or down) when going just up or just down.

| Great pyramid 1 Complete 3 sets of the pyramid and then rest* | | | | Great pyramid 2 Complete 3 sets of the pyramid and then rest* | | | |
|---|---|---|---|---|---|---|---|
| Exercise | Reps for set 1 | Reps for set 2 | Reps for set 3 | Exercise | Reps for set 1 | Reps for set 2 | Reps for set 3 |
| Leg press | 15-20 | 10-15 | 6-10 | Squat | 15-20 | 10-15 | 6-10 |
| Bent-over barbell row | 15-20 | 10-15 | 6-10 | Lat pull-down | 15-20 | 10-15 | 6-10 |
| Bench press | 15-20 | 10-15 | 6-10 | Dumbbell incline bench press | 15-20 | 10-15 | 6-10 |
| Lateral raise | 15-20 | 10-15 | 6-10 | Barbell shoulder press | 15-20 | 10-15 | 6-10 |
| Straight bar curl | 15-20 | 10-15 | 6-10 | Supine triceps extension | 15-20 | 10-15 | 6-10 |
| Dumbbell triceps extension | 15-20 | 10-15 | 6-10 | E-Z bar preacher curl | 15-20 | 10-15 | 6-10 |
| | Rest 60 sec. | Rest 90 sec. | Rest 2 min. | | Rest 60 sec. | Rest 90 sec. | Rest 2 min. |

*Experienced lifters can perform a 4th set using only the first 3 exercises in each pyramid. Complete 2 to 6 reps per exercise for this set, and take 2 min. rest.

# Preexhaust or Postexhaust Routine

In this challenging routine, perform 10 to 12 repetitions of the first exercise and 8 to 10 of the second, with no rest between each pair. For the triple exhaust, switch to the third exercise and perform 6 to 8 reps, again with no break, before taking your break in between each set. You may alternate upper and lower body exercises or perform the upper, then the lower. Perform one or two sets of each pair or trio. More than two sets is not necessary because, if executed properly, you will get a very good workout, as your total volume is already doubled. Be careful on the triple exhaust—it is not easy, and fatigue sets in fast. Be prepared to decrease the weight you would normally use for these exercises.

| Double exhaust | | | |
|---|---|---|---|
| Preexhaust Rest 90 sec. between pairs | | Postexhaust Rest 90 sec. between pairs | |
| Exercise | Reps | Exercise | Reps |
| Dumbbell pec fly* | 10-12 | Bench press | 10-12 |
| Bench press | 8-10 | Dumbbell pec fly* | 8-10 |
| Leg extension | 10-12 | Leg press | 10-12 |
| Leg press | 8-10 | Leg extension | 8-10 |
| Dumbbell pullover | 10-12 | Lat pull-down | 10-12 |
| Lat pull-down | 8-10 | Dumbbell pullover | 8-10 |
| Heel raise | 10-12 | Lying leg curl | 10-12 |
| Lying leg curl | 8-10 | Heel raise | 8-10 |
| Supine triceps extension | 10-12 | Shoulder press | 10-12 |
| Shoulder press | 8-10 | Lateral raise | 8-10 |
| Crunch | 10-12 | Crunch | 10-12 |
| Back extension | 8-10 | Back extension | 8-10 |

| Triple exhaust | | | |
|---|---|---|---|
| **Preexhaust** Rest 90 sec. between trios | | **Postexhaust** Rest 90 sec. between trios | |
| **Exercise** | **Reps** | **Exercise** | **Reps** |
| Dumbbell pec fly* | 10-12 | Bench press | 10-12 |
| Bench press | 8-10 | Dumbbell pec fly* | 8-10 |
| Cable cross | 6-8 | Incline bench press | 6-8 |
| Leg extension | 10-12 | Leg press | 10-12 |
| Leg press | 8-10 | Leg extension | 8-10 |
| Leg extension | 6-8 | Leg press | 6-8 |
| Dumbbell pullover | 10-12 | Lat pull-down | 10-12 |
| Lat pull-down | 8-10 | Dumbbell pullover | 8-10 |
| Dumbbell pullover | 6-8 | Lat pull-down | 6-8 |
| Heel raise | 10-12 | Lying leg curl | 10-12 |
| Lying leg curl | 8-10 | Heel raise | 8-10 |
| Seated calf heel raise | 6-8 | Seated leg curl | 6-8 |
| Supine triceps extension | 10-12 | Shoulder press | 10-12 |
| Shoulder press | 8-10 | Lateral raise | 8-10 |
| Supine triceps extension | 6-8 | Shoulder press | 6-8 |
| Crunch | 10-12 | Crunch | 10-12 |
| Back extension | 8-10 | Back extension | 8-10 |

*The machine pec fly may be done instead of the dumbbell pec fly.

# Dumbbell Circuits

Dumbbell circuits are perfect to perform in a busy gym or at home if you have a few dumbbells and a bench. For each exercise, select dumbbells you can perform 12 to 15 reps with. Perform each exercise in the circuit with little or no rest in between. Beginners should do one or two circuits, resting three minutes between each; advanced lifters may take shorter rests and perform as many as five circuits. Make sure you emphasize good technique even as you fatigue. Circuits can be done two or three nonconsecutive days per week.

| **Beginner circuit** 12-15 reps per exercise | **Intermediate circuit** 12-15 reps per exercise | **Advanced circuit** 12-15 reps per exercise |
|---|---|---|
| Squat | Lunge | Lunge |
| Dumbbell bench press | Dumbbell row | Dumbbell Romanian deadlift |
| Dumbbell row | Dumbbell incline bench press | Alternating dumbbell bench press |
| Lateral raise | Dumbbell shoulder press | Dumbbell row |
| Isolated dumbbell curl | Dumbbell triceps kickback | Front raise and lateral raise |
| Supine triceps extension | Hammer curl | Overhead triceps extension Dumbbell curl |
| Rest 3 min. | Rest 3 min. | Rest 3 min. |

# SPLIT ROUTINES

Splits are the most popular way to work out. They are more challenging and help isolate specific areas. For the split to be effective, you should work out at least two times a week. Advanced bodybuilders may work out as many as six times a week, but to stay safe and prevent overtraining, don't plan more than four weight training sessions a week. With split routines, you need to rest your muscles 24 to 48 hours before you work the same group of muscles again.

## Two-Day Repeat

This workout is designed for the person who likes to work out and challenge the body to work overtime. Day 1 and day 2 are repeated again later in the week, so you will perform each routine twice during a week. Additionally, twice a week you will add leg work on either day 1 or day 2, but not both.

| Day 1<br>Rest 2 min. after each of the first 4 exercises and then 90 sec. after each of the other exercises | | | Day 2<br>Rest 2 min. after each of the first 4 exercises and then 90 sec. after each of the other exercises | | |
|---|---|---|---|---|---|
| Push exercise | Sets | Reps | Pull exercise | Sets | Reps |
| Bench press | 3 | 8 | Seated row | 3 | 8 |
| Incline bench press | 3 | 8 | Lat pull-down | 3 | 8 |
| Shoulder press | 2 | 8 | Lat pull-down (palms turned in) | 2 | 8 |
| Dip | 2 | 10 | Straight bar curl | 2 | 10 |
| Machine pec fly | 2 | 10 | Preacher curl | 2 | 10 |
| Supine triceps extension | 2 | 10 | Dumbbell curl | 2 | 10 |
| Triceps push-down | 2 | 10 | Crunch | 3 | 12 |
| Lateral raise | 2 | 10 | | | |
| **Leg workout for day 1 or day 2**<br>Rest 2 min. after each of the first 3 exercises and then 90 sec. after each of the other exercises | | | | | |
| Exercise | | Sets | | Reps | |
| Leg press | | 3 | | 8-12 | |
| Leg extension | | 3 | | 8-12 | |
| Lying leg curl | | 3 | | 8-12 | |
| Heel raise | | 3 | | 8-12 | |

## Four-Day Supersplit

The following routine is a traditional bodybuilding split. If you have four days to work out each week for at least four weeks, this routine will make you look great. It focuses on individual body parts, getting everything covered within a week and still giving you time to live your normal life. Even beginners can do this one because there is adequate rest time. Advanced lifters can increase the number of sets, while beginners can perform one or two sets of each exercise. In between workout days, take a much-needed rest, as the goal is to push as hard as possible on those days you are working out.

| Day 1 | Day 2 | Day 3 | Day 4 |
|---|---|---|---|
| Complete 3 sets of 10-12 reps for each exercise Rest 90 sec. after each set | | Complete 3-4 sets of 8-10 reps for each exercise Rest 75 sec. after each set | |
| Dumbbell Incline bench press | Leg press | Bench press | Single-leg press |
| Dumbbell bench press | Leg press | Incline bench press | Lunge |
| Dumbbell incline pec fly | Seated leg curl | Cable cross | Single-leg curl |
| Dumbbell shoulder press | Heel raise | Machine pec fly | Seated calf heel raise |
| Shoulder shrug | Dumbbell row | Machine shoulder press | Wide-grip lat pull-down |
| Supine triceps extension | Close-grip lat pull-down | Overhead triceps extension | Lat pull-down (palms turned in) |
| Triceps push-down | Straight-arm lat pull-down | Cable reverse-grip triceps pull-down | Machine seated row |
| Crunch | E-Z bar preacher curl | Twisting crunch | Cable curl |
| Twisting crunch | Barbell biceps curl | Plank | Alternating dumbbell curl |

# CHALLENGE YOURSELF

If you get bored with your usual routine, try one of the following programs to add variety and provide a challenge. They are specific routines with a given set of instructions. Of course, these routines can be modified to fit your needs or your imagination.

Several of these routines are specific to target those weak areas. Although the general rule of thumb is to start with the larger muscle groups and progress down to the smaller ones, if you have a particularly weak area or just want to make a certain part of your body better, you have to target train. Don't be afraid—we all want to look good, and target training is the way to get there. Even though spot reduction of fat is impossible, you can definitely tighten the muscles in a particular area, so even that extra fat may look a little better.

## Bad to the Core

Perhaps one of the most overrated body parts is the abdominal region. Without trimming the fat, no exercise on this planet will help you achieve the six-pack look. But a solid foundation of core work, including both your back and abs, will help reduce injury, improve posture, and improve overall health. But more important, you can brag later about how hard you trained your core, which is the new buzz word when it comes to exercise.

| Day 1 Rest 90-120 sec. between sets | | | Day 2 Rest 90-120 sec. between sets | | |
|---|---|---|---|---|---|
| Exercise | Sets | Reps | Exercise | Sets | Reps |
| Plank | 3 | 8 | Elbow to hand plank lift | 3 | 8 |
| Lateral plank raise | 2 | 10 | Lateral plank raise | 2 | 10 |
| Fire hydrant | 2 | 12 | Rotational fire hydrant | 2 | 12 |
| Back extension | 2 | 12 | Back extension | 2 | 12 |
| Crunch | 3 | 15 | Reverse crunch | 3 | 15 |
| Pelvic raise | 2 | 10 | Standing rotational twist | 3 | 10 |
| Side bends | 2 | 10 each side | Stability ball leg curl | 3 | 10 |
| Axe chops | 2 | 12 | | | |

## Reach Your Peak

Everybody wants bigger or well-toned arms. The peak workout will increase size and definition in both the biceps and triceps, giving your arms the appearance you've always wanted. This workout should be performed a maximum of two times per week. Sets should be taken to or near muscular failure. Using short rest intervals (around 60 seconds) between sets will maximize growth. Don't neglect the other muscle groups in the body while doing this workout. Make sure you perform leg, back, chest, and core work at least once during the week.

| Beginner Complete 10-12 reps per set Rest 60 sec. between sets | | Intermediate Complete 10-12 reps per set Rest 60 sec. between sets | | Advanced Complete 10-12 reps per set Rest 60 sec. between sets | |
|---|---|---|---|---|---|
| Exercise | Sets | Exercise | Sets | Exercise | Sets |
| Dumbbell curl | 2 | Barbell biceps curl | 3 | E-Z bar preacher curl and dumbbell curl | 3 supersets |
| Triceps push-down | 2 | E-Z bar preacher curl | 2 | Barbell biceps curl | 3 |
| Cable curl | 2 | Dumbbell isolation curl | 2 | Cable curl | 3 |
| Dumbbell triceps kickback | 2 | Overhead triceps extension | 3 | Supine triceps extension and bench dip | 3 supersets |
| Hammer curl | 2 | Triceps push-down | 2 | Triceps push-down | 3 |
| Bench dip | 2 | Cable reverse-grip triceps push-down | 2 | Overhead triceps extension | 3 |

# Build the Base

By the name, it sounds like a sheer mass builder. Ladies, don't be scared; for you, it will be more of a leg and butt toner while making sure your lower back and abs get some good work. The key is to push yourself with heavy weights rather than take a circuit-style approach with minimal rest and lighter weights.

| Day 1 Rest 2-3 min. between set | | | Day 2 Rest 2-3 min. between set | | |
|---|---|---|---|---|---|
| Exercise | Sets | Reps | Exercise | Sets | Reps |
| Squat | 3 | 8 | Single-leg squat | 3 | 8 each leg |
| Step-up | 2 | 10 | Dumbbell squat | 2 | 15 |
| Lunge | 3 | 10 each leg | Walking lunge | 3 | 8 each leg |
| Straight-leg deadlift | 2 | 8 | Single-leg extension | 2 | 12 |
| Leg curl (depending on what they have at their gym) | 3 | 12 | Stability ball leg curl | 3 | 10 |
| Heel raise | 2 | 10 | Single-leg heel raise | 2 | 12 each leg |
| Seated calf heel raise | 2 | 10 | Single-leg heel raise | 2 | 12 each leg |
| Crunch | 3 | 12-15 | Twisting crunch | 3 | 12-15 |
| Back extension | 3 | 12-15 | Back extension | 3 | 12-15 |

# Leg-Acy

This routine will leave a lasting impression. Repeat this program at least twice if not three times. When you finish, your legs will feel like jelly, making it hard for you to stand. If not, repeat for another round! Continue reps until failure, and always use perfect technique.

| No.* | Supersets** | Reps | Notes | Rest after superset |
|------|-------------|------|-------|---------------------|
| 1 | Leg extension<br>Seated leg curl | 10<br>10 | For each rep, count 1 sec. up and 2 sec. down | 90 sec. |
| 2 | Leg extension<br>Seated leg curl | 5<br>5 | Use 1/2 to 3/4 the weight used in set 1<br>For each rep, count 5 sec. up, hold 5 sec., and count 5 sec. down<br>Maintain form and time for the entire set | 90 sec. |
| 3 | Leg extension<br>Seated leg curl | 6<br>6 | Use 1 1/4 to 1 1/2 times the weight used in set 1<br>Negative training: spotter lifts weight to top position, and lifter lowers it using a 4 count | 3 min. |
| 4 | Adductor cable lift<br>Side cable lift<br>Hip Extension***<br>Lunge | 12<br>12<br>12<br>12 each leg | For each rep, count 2 sec. up and 3 sec. down | 2 min. |
| 5 | Lunge<br>Adductor cable lift<br>Side cable lift<br>Hip Extension*** | 12<br>12<br>12<br>12 | For each rep, count 2 sec. up and 3 sec. down | 3 min. |
| 6 | Heel raise<br>Seated calf heel raise | 10<br>10 | For each rep, count 2 sec. up and 3 sec. down<br>If you do not reach failure at the 10th rep, use more weight | 30-60 sec. |
| 7 | Heel raise<br>Seated calf heel raise | 10<br>10 | For each rep, count 2 sec. up and 3 sec. down<br>If you do not reach failure at the 10th rep, use more weight | 30-60s |

*If you need the work, repeat either the 4th or 5th set. If you need more calf work, you can repeat the 6th and 7th supersets.
**Do not rest between the exercises in each superset.
***If a good hip extension machine is not available, perform a cable hip extension in its place.

## Butt and Thigh Blaster

All ladies getting ready for bathing suit season know all too well the objective of this workout: to hammer the butt and thighs for some serious toning (with the aid of a little fat loss too, of course). The butt and thigh blaster workout can be performed by people of any training status; however, beginners should not train to failure and should perform the workout only one or two days per week (separated by at least 72 hours). More advanced trainees can consider performing this workout up to three times per week, provided muscle soreness is not excessive. Rest intervals should be kept short, around 60 to 75 seconds between sets.

| Beginner workout<br>Rest 60-75 sec. between sets | | | Intermediate workout<br>Rest 60-75 sec. between sets | | | Advanced workout<br>Rest 60-75 sec. between sets | | |
|---|---|---|---|---|---|---|---|---|
| Exercise | Sets | Reps | Exercise | Sets | Reps | Exercise | Sets | Reps |
| Hip extension | 2 | 12-15 | Hip extension | 2 | 12-15 | Hip extension | 3 | 12-15 |
| Lying leg curl | 3 | 10-12 | Single-leg curl | 3 | 10-12 | Straight-leg deadlift | 3 | 8-12 |
| Leg press | 3 | 8-10 | Single-leg press | 3 | 8-10 | Step-up | 3 | 8-10 |
| Side-cable lift | 2 | 12-15 | Squat<br>Body-weight squat | 2 supersets | 10 reps per exercise | Leg press (1 leg at a time) | 3 | 10-12 |
| Adductor cable lift | 2 | 12-15 | | | | Walking lunge | 2 | 20 each leg |
| | | | | | | Body-weight squat | 2 | 20 |

## Tug o' War

This routine is a push–pull nightmare that will leave you exhausted without the rope burn. Designed primarily to build strength, athletes will do this for several circuits; however, for a solid upper body burn, anyone can do this workout.

| No. | Exercise | Reps | Notes | Rest |
|---|---|---|---|---|
| 1 | Bench press<br>Seated row<br>Shoulder press<br>Lat pull-down<br>Triceps push-down<br>Cable curl | 6<br>6<br>6<br>6<br>6<br>6 | Begin with a weight with which you can perform 10 reps<br>For each rep, count 2 sec. up, hold for 4 sec., and count 2 sec. down | 3 min. |
| 2 | Bench press<br>Seated row<br>Shoulder press<br>Lat pull-down<br>Triceps push-down<br>Cable curl | 6<br>6<br>6<br>6<br>6<br>6 | Use 2/3 the weight used in set 1<br>For each rep, count 2 sec. up, hold 4 sec., and count 2 sec. down | 2 min. |
| 3 | Bench press<br>Seated row<br>Shoulder press<br>Lat pull-down<br>Triceps push-down<br>Cable curl | 6<br>6<br>6<br>6<br>6<br>6 | Use 2/3 the weight used in set 2<br>For each rep, count 2 sec. up, hold 4 sec., and count 2 sec. down | Rest 3 min.<br>Repeat this set<br>Rest 5 min. |
| 4 | Dumbbell pec fly<br>Dumbbell bench press | 10<br>10 | This superset will exhaust the muscle going into set 5, so choose your weight carefully | 60 sec. |
| 5 | Rear deltoid fly<br>Dumbbell row | 10<br>10 | This superset will exhaust the muscle going into set 6, so choose your weight carefully | 60 sec. |
| 6 | Dumbbell triceps kickback<br>Dumbbell curl | 10<br>10 | Your muscles should feel a bit fatigued by now, so choose your weight carefully and go for it! | Rest 3 min.<br>Repeat sets 4, 5, and 6 |

# Dumbbell Complex

Dumbbells are a great way to add variation to your routine. The movement is the same, although you will need to watch your form and keep your body stable. Immediately move through each exercise, taking only 30 seconds' rest before moving to the next one. As you continue through this routine, you will probably need to increase your rest time. Don't let this one fool you—it is a truly challenging routine. This supercircuit pulls out all the stops.

| First circuit<br>**Perform 12 reps of each exercise**<br>Rest 30 sec. between exercises | Second circuit<br>**Perform 12 reps of each exercise**<br>Rest 30 sec. between exercises | Third circuit: supersets*<br>**Perform 12 reps of each exercise**<br>Rest 30 sec. between supersets |
|---|---|---|
| Dumbbell bench press | Dumbbell bench press | Squat (dumbbells held at shoulders)<br>Dumbbell shoulder press |
| Dumbbell row | Squat (dumbbells held at shoulders) | Dumbbell straight-leg deadlift<br>Dumbbell upright row |
| Dumbbell shoulder press | Dumbbell row | Dumbbell bench press<br>Dumbbell triceps kickback or overhead extension |
| Dumbbell upright row | Dumbbell straight-leg deadlift | Dumbbell row<br>Dumbbell curl |
| Dumbbell triceps kickback or overhead triceps extension | Dumbbell shoulder press | Single-leg heel raise (dumbbells hanging at sides)<br>Crunch (dumbbells held at shoulders) |
| Dumbbell curl | Single-leg heel raise (dumbbells hanging at sides) | |
| Squats (dumbbells held at shoulders) | Dumbbell upright row | |
| Dumbbell straight-leg deadlift | Crunch (dumbbells held at shoulders) | |
| Single-leg heel raise (dumbbells hanging at sides) | Dumbbell triceps kickback or overhead triceps extension | |
| Crunch (dumbbells held at shoulders) | Dumbbell curl | |

*Perform the first set of the first movement, and then perform the first set of the second movement before taking a rest.

# ABOUT THE AUTHOR

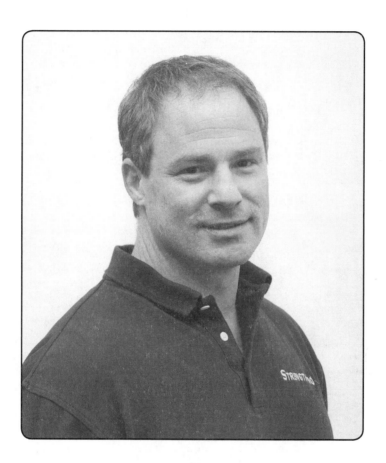

**David Sandler** has served as science advisor for Spike TV's *Jesse James Is a Dead Man* series, Fox Sports' *Sport Science* series, and National Geographic's *Fight Science, Super Strength, The Science of Steroids,* and *Humanly Possible* shows. He is president and cofounder of StrengthPro Inc. and a member of the advisory boards for *Muscle and Fitness Magazine, Muscle Mag International, Reps, Maximum Fitness,* and *Performance Training Journal of the NSCA*.

Sandler has been a strength and conditioning consultant for two decades and presented at almost 300 lectures worldwide with organizations such as the NSCA, ACSM, AFPA, AAHPERD, IFPA, SWIS, ECA, and SCW Fitness. He was the recipient of the Faculty of the Year Award in 2005 for the International Fitness Professionals Association (IFPA).

Sandler has also authored or coauthored 5 books, over 20 scientific articles, and more than 150 articles in power and strength training magazines, including *Muscle and Fitness, Men's Health,* and *Oxygen*. As a former world-class powerlifter, Sandler focuses his research in strength and power development.

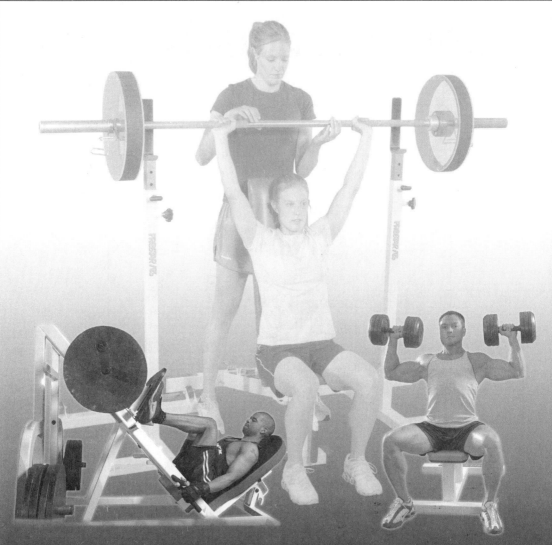